Dear Aman[illegible]

&

Noah

May you read c̄ love

as it is written c̄

Love

Remi

AYURVEDA
TO THE RESCUE

AN ANCIENT REMEDY FOR MODERN AILMENTS

Renu Chaudhary

First Edition – March 2014

ISBN
978-1-4602-3434-1 (Hardcover)
978-1-4602-3435-8 (Paperback)
978-1-4602-3436-5 (eBook)

Front cover illustration by Socrates Genes
for more information please visit www.sacredgates.com
Flow chart illustration and Tongue diagram: organ vs tastes
are copyright works by Dr. Vasant Lad of The Ayurvedic Institute.

Produced by:

FriesenPress
Suite 300 – 852 Fort Street
Victoria, BC, Canada V8W 1H8

www.friesenpress.com

Distributed to the trade by The Ingram Book Company

Contents

Author's Note

Millions of books have been written thus far on Ayurveda, so why one more?

Over the years, my yearning to write about Ayurveda in the context of modern-day life and to share its relevance in these challenging times has become stronger and stronger. Today we need to welcome back Ayurveda so it can reclaim its glory and rightful place in our modern health-care systems.

Those around me encouraged me, and so trusting my innermost calling, I gave birth to this tribute to Ayurveda, one of my greatest passions in life. Made of two root words – "ayur" meaning "life" and "veda" meaning "knowledge", Ayurveda is the knowledge of life itself. Hence came about *Ayurveda to the Rescue: An Ancient Remedy for Modern Ailments.*

Ayurveda has surrounded each aspect of my life. Nothing exists outside of its scope. By sharing it with you, I hope its wisdom embraces you all as it has embraced me for the past three decades of this life.

My goal is to write about its relevance in everyday, simple ways without going in to the intellectual symbolism of this knowledge. For that, there are millions of other great texts available. I am choosing to use simple language that focuses on the basics in order to reach the most average reader and earnest aspirant. However, the most inquisitive of minds may yearn to learn more. If this stirs and triggers in you a thirst to know more, my efforts have been successful in bringing the valuable benefits of this complete spiritual healing science to you.

I am thankful that recent events have allowed the birth of this project to become a reality. May the "Master's Grace" shine through this and shower you the reader. Without this "Grace" none is possible and with this "Grace" nothing is impossible.

Lovingly,

Karunakshie

Editor's Note

Ayurveda to the Rescue is an in-depth examination of Ayurveda, an ancient science and a complete wellness modality around healing and staying healthy. Covering both the theoretical and practical aspects of this ancient wisdom, this book makes a comprehensive guide for the beginner wishing to learn about Ayurveda. As the author notes: "Today, health is defined only as absence of life-threatening diseases and gives next to no importance to living a balanced, healthy lifestyle." This book will help to correct this.

This book's greatest strength is the wealth of information it provides. The author covers both the theoretical and practical sides of Ayurveda so that readers can understand and appreciate the reasons for the practices introduced. There is a tremendous amount of information presented in this book, but it is accessible because it is presented in a clear, logical progression of ideas – starting with the history and rationale of Ayurveda and concluding with practical information on diet.

Another strength is the many comprehensive tables and lists included in the book with useful information on such things as "Tastes vs. Part of Tongue vs. Organs" and "Ghritas" (medicated herbal Ghee) vs. Benefits vs. Herb Usage".

E. Siegel, Writer/Editor/Researcher

Book Reviews

I have had the great fortune of having Ayurvedic consultations with Renu Chaudhary, who is an exceptional Ayurvedic therapist. I began to realize that I had finally found a true healer whose understanding of health was not just about the body, but also about mind and spirit. She taught me that these three things contribute to living in this world in a healthy, whole way.

This book, *Ayurveda to the Rescue: An Ancient Remedy for Modern Ailments*, will get you back onto the road to good health. The valuable information on these pages offers an invitation to the whole life. This book is a collection of factual knowledge with wisdom of tradition and compassionate intuition that blends medicine with spirit in humanity's abode. The information in this book gives us a foothold to understanding what it means to live as a consciously whole human being.

Many of us are aware that we have lost our way to good health, and because of this, we are searching for answers to improve and keep our good health. This book shows us how to do that. We are in need of this ancient medicine that has proven itself for more than five thousand years. People are searching for a more natural way of living and healing their whole being, and because of that, Ayurvedic medicine is becoming well known globally and has become a much sought after healing modality.

We are not all the same, and Ayurvedic medicine takes all that into consideration. When we are ill, we just think about healing our body – but we are not just our bodies, we are so much more than that. All parts must work together as a whole for good health on all levels. Ayurvedic medicine deals with all of these modalities, and a perfect health plan is created.

This book will help you to restore your body, mind, and soul. You will learn to create a diet for you alone based on foods that will lead to clarity, calmness, peace, and good health.

Carole Davis, MA,
Editor of *Wake Up!*
Vedic Astrologer
1-888-406-9668

—

Ayurveda has been in practice for thousands of years in India. The art of Ayurveda lies in the use of nutrition and herbs. These are pivotal in a healing that is tailored to an individual's genetic makeup.

Renu Chaudhary is a qualified Ayurvedic practitioner whom I have known for many years. She is a spiritual individual who is very passionate about nutrition and health. This book is her tribute to that passion of hers.

Ayurveda to the Rescue consists of Ayurvedic concepts that are easy to grasp and apply in day-to-day practice. I highly recommend this book as a daily read for the enhancement of an individual's nutritional health.

This book will help you to understand "who you are" and how you can get to know yourself in mind, body, and spirit.

The cover's beauty is worth a thousand words. The tables, flow chart, and diagrams will help the reader to visualize the practical aspects in simple ways.

As food is the music of love, let us eat well!

Dr. Verandra P. Jivan M.D.

—

I have known Renu Chaudhary for the last two decades – both as a friend and as my personal Ayurvedic consultant. I knew that she is a remarkable woman, but did not know about her remarkable abilities in writing until I started reading her book, which is now ready to go into the hands of thousands of readers. It is a topic that well-known authors like Dr. Vasant Lad and Dr. Deepak Chopra have introduced to millions all over the world.

What is unique about this new book, *Ayurveda to the Rescue,* is that it is easily read, and abstract concepts are clearly explained. Reading this book makes me feel as if my dear Ayurveda mentor is sitting by my side, helping me to resolve my dilemmas in the healing process.

Renu Chaudhary has also provided an experiential tour of daily practices and tips, which are not so quickly available in other treatises on this subject. I am sure that this will be one of the very few books and standards in my kitchen cabinet and will continue to have a real impact on my life.

It will add years to my life and life to my years, and I bless that it will do the same to many others around the globe!

Raju Ramanathan P.Eng
Voting member, US Technical Advisory Group to ISO/TC 176

—

Dear Renu Karunakshi

I know you have a great talent for making your points concise and readable. You express yourself clearly and convey using ancient, eastern perspective to the modern minds. Let this book open a window on your apparent ideas of the life of the real yogi's of the east. I know You are a joyful person, intensely involved person and can present the deepest concepts most lucidly.

Lots of love and blessings to you.
Amma

If you gather the whole world in your accumulation ,you will still feel insufficient as there is something within you which will not settle for any thing because its nature is that of the creator himself.

Param Poojya Gurumatha Amma
Spiritual Master
Sridharagudda
Kengeri , India

Dedications and Gratitude

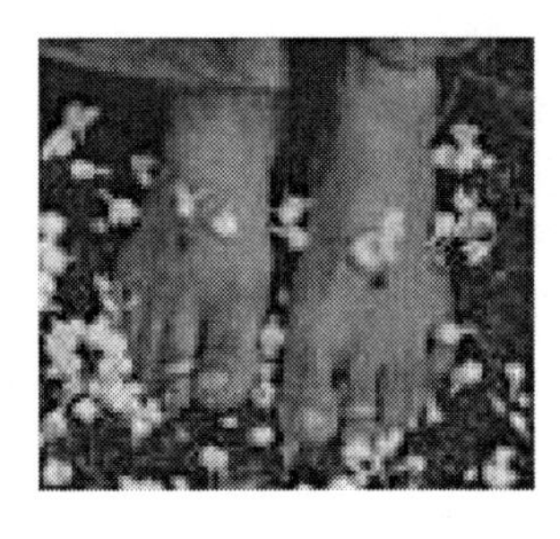

This work is dedicated to all the Masters who have touched my life and guided me through my journey of self-discovery. Without their input, I would be perpetually lost. I remain eternally grateful for their trust and grace to even attempt to compile this work. I dedicate it all at their lotus feet!

To my maternal grandmother, whose culinary skills were simple and exceptional, it seems I owe her the gift of my culinary passions.

To my Parents, without whom, I would not be here to learn about myself. To them I am forever grateful for gifting me a body. It then became a vehicle through which to experience life and to explore the beauty of the true grace of the mind, which is hosted by the equally wonderful soul.

To my soul mate, best friend, and husband "Karunesh", whose support has been a pillar of strength in my life. Without him, nothing would have mattered.

To all my children, for giving me ample opportunities to learn about life and to expand my heart beyond what I thought I could possibly do. To my siblings, for all your support and love for me no matter what I asked of you all. Today I honour you all for your individual uniqueness, which I have come to understand and realize, while I thank you all for accepting me with my limitations. Truth always mattered to me the most. To my grandchildren, who are showing me it was all worth it.

To Bela, my dearest one, for your patience, diligent support, and standing up to my unending demands to read and approve and re-read my material at insane hours of day and night, I salute you.

To all the challenges that became treasures of learning about myself, I remain deeply grateful for the opportunities they presented. To my limitations, for without seeing them I would have never embarked upon my journey of self-discovery for which I am ever grateful.

To my friends, who have been as numerous as they are unique, for adding their own colour to my life.

To the beings of this planet, who have crossed my path and enriched my life in more ways than I can mention – and this encompasses plants, animals, and humans alike! For the love of Nature and its silent teachings, I am earnestly and humbly grateful!

Chapter One

The Ancient Wisdom: A Gift To Humankind

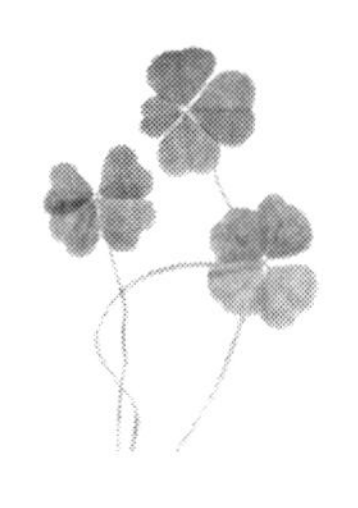

"The Science of life shall never attain finality. Therefore, humility and relentless industry should characterize your endeavour and your approach to knowledge. The entire world consists of teachers for the wise and enemies for the fools. Therefore, knowledge, conducive to health, longevity, fame, and excellence, coming from even an unknown source, should be received, assimilated, and utilized with earnestness."

—Charaka Samhita

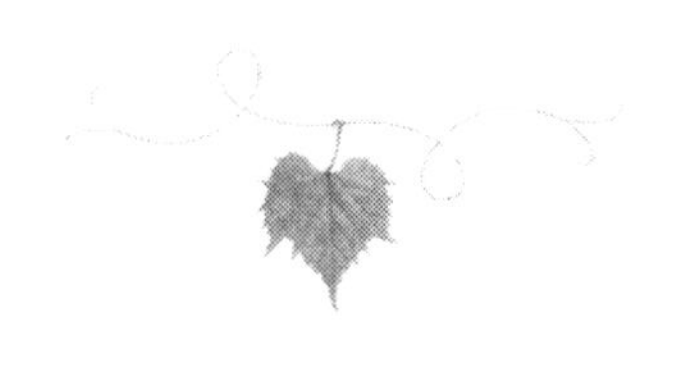

Ancient Wisdom: Its Relevance in Modern Times

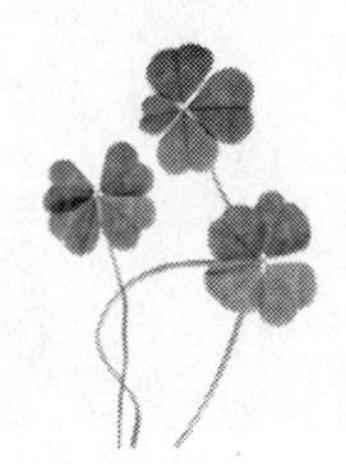

Ayurveda, an ancient wisdom of healing science, is not just a health-care system, but a holistic, preventive healing modality immersed in a centuries old proven science. It is relevant in its practical manner of living life tuned to the rhythms of nature. Today, humankind has gone far from its natural roots in the name of technological progress. The human race has paid a tremendous price for this error of omission in the name of technological advancements. In these modern times, humankind is facing more illnesses than enjoying the joys of simple health.

People today are more interested in taking charge of their own healing in their own hands. This is an attempt to make the ancient wisdom available to the humans of today. Truth has the power to prevail through changing times without losing its efficacy and relevance. Language should not be a barrier in accessing this treasure. Therefore, simplicity is used to bring the essence of Ayurveda into a modern-day context for you.

Ayurveda is the symbiosis of two Sanskrit words: "ayur" meaning "life" and "veda" meaning knowledge. It is, therefore, the knowledge of life itself. It is potently immersed in knowledge of total well-being. Totality is its strength and deliverance is its gift to humankind.

Knowledge can only render its true essence when applied. Life is cyclic: what is born today will live for a little while, then decay and die. This is life's very nature. But one who dies while living entails a true awakening. True Awakening is awaiting us. Ayurveda has in its bosom all that is needed to unfold the many layers of your own reality. It is a simple, clear, concise, and meticulously accurate science, philosophy, and spirituality all blended into one. If it is followed with true reverence and devotion to self, one can reap its countless benefits.

This is the journey of a lifetime, and it takes a lifetime to unfold. There are neither shortcuts to health, nor easy quick fixes. As humans, we only take on something if we see its importance in our daily existence. Having said this, your due patience and healthy sense of self-worth will aid you as you continue this journey that begins with one step. It is not a part-time endeavour that one can take on and expect quick results. Rather, it is a process that will continue to unfold your own truth to you. You are worth the effort. You are worth this indulgence. Make the choice now and follow through without focusing on the outcome. The outcome will present itself in due course of time and the joy of true health will kiss your feet.

Old is Gold

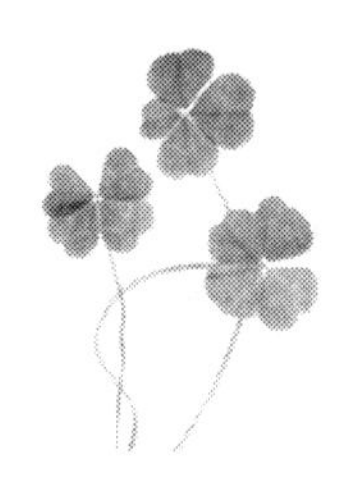

Ayurveda belongs to and is mentioned in the oldest ancient Hindu Holy Scriptures known as the *Vedas*[1]. The origin of the Vedas dates back 5000 years. It finds a special mention in the *Atharva Veda,*[2] which includes instructions on how humankind should live respecting the natural cycles in order to remain healthy, wealthy, and wise.

As the story of humankind progressed, less and less importance was given to simple natural cycles. Soon, they were replaced with shortcut methods of modern-day living. Today we are close to totally forgetting that "old is gold". This "gold" must be preserved in order to survive changing times and changing needs of the time. Modern-day humans need to wake up to its importance and its relevance in day-to-day existence.

---

1 "Vedas" come from the root word "veda", meaning "knowledge and teachings". Vedas are the ancient scriptures of India, containing this knowledge. There are four Vedas: Rig Veda, Sama Veda, Yajur Veda, and Atharva Veda.

2 Atharva Veda is the fourth of the four Vedas, outlining the every-day protocols of how one must live aligned with nature. Ayur-veda is considered Upa-veda of the Atharva veda; simply meaning the "cream essence" of the Atharva Veda.

Today health is defined only as the absence of life-threatening diseases and gives next to no importance to living a balanced, healthy lifestyle. *No medicine can cure the damage caused by disregarding the inner intelligence with which we are gifted.* This ancient wisdom personifies the importance of the natural forces and changing rhythms; hence, daily and seasonal changes entail changing lifestyles. Our ancestors knew this and lived surrounded by this wisdom.

Modern-day humans are now left with no choice but to go back to the basics of when humankind prospered equally and lived in perfect harmony respecting the natural forces of nature.

Today we have more illnesses and even more pharmaceutical solutions, which due to their efficacy, have totally diluted the need for maintaining a healthy life style. *No medicine can compensate for unhealthy living.*

Ayurvedic principles are timeless knowledge, and therefore the core principles' validity continues to be effective even today if used with total trust, respect, and devotion. Ayurveda comes from the one of most ancient literary works known to humankind. It was orally transmitted by "God himself'" to those who were in *higher states of consciousness.* The oral instructions were bestowed upon selected aspirants who were ardently tuned to finding deeper secrets within themselves to lead a complete life at all three dimensions of human existence.

We must keep in mind that a human is not just a physical form having a spiritual experience, but rather a spiritual being having a human experience. Therefore, we must honour all its three aspects – the physical, mental, and spiritual dimensions – for a total human existence. The time has come, and we must reclaim our birthright to live a holistically healthy and emotionally fulfilling life. Propagating this wisdom globally to a modern mindset will ensure its survival. Ayurveda was, Ayurveda is, and Ayurveda will continue to be. The question to ask is: Are we ready to join in its exploration, time and time again?

The time to re-visit and re-explore this ancient gift has arrived. The time is NOW HERE. We must stand up to these challenging times equipped with the oldest remedial gift available to us; one that is as fresh today as the day it was born.

Chapter Two

The Birth Of Ayurveda: The Theory of Creation

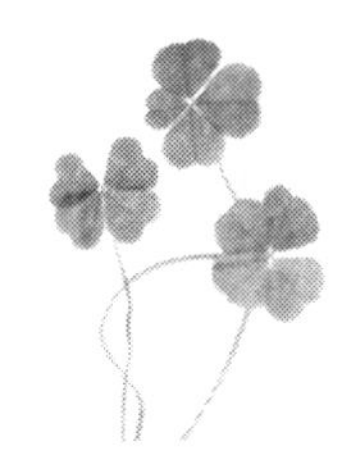

"There is no end to learning Ayurveda. You should carefully and constantly devote yourself to its study. Increase your skill by learning from others without jealousy. The wise regard the whole world as their teacher, while the ignorant consider it to be their enemy."

—Charaka

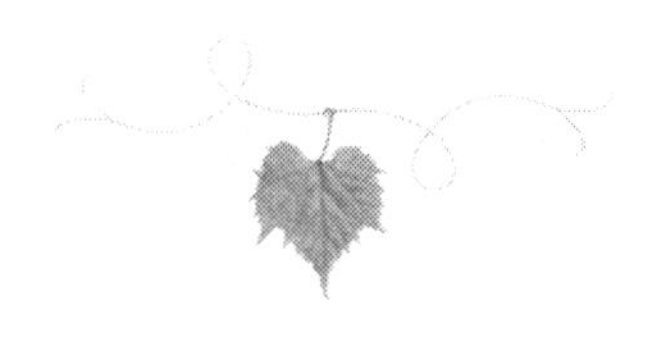

Theory of Creation: "The Sankhya Philosophy"

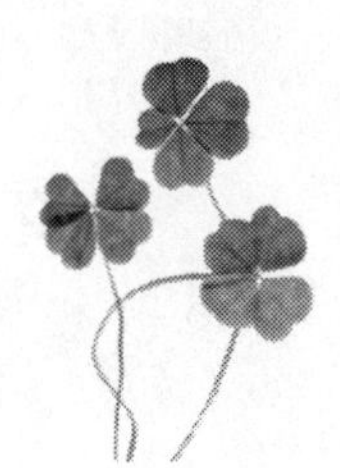

Ayurveda is the oldest known written text available to humankind, dating back approximately 5000 years. Its origin is the very point of time when consciousness itself yearned to express itself through the union of the male and the female energies present in our cosmic space.

Ayurveda incorporates the Six Systems of Indian Philosophy namely: *Sankhya,*[3] *Nyaya,*[4] *Vaisheshika,*[5] *Mimamsa,*[6] *Yoga,*[7] *and Vedanta.*[8] The six systems symbolize "Shad-Dharshana"; "shad" meaning "six" and "Dharshana" meaning "to see". These six philosophies are accepted and propagated by Ayurveda for the total healing of humankind.

The first three philosophies – Sankhya, Nyaya, and Vaisheshika – help us to understand our physical universe. The theory of creation enumerated

---

3 Sankhya is a Sanskrit word meaning "enumeration". Sage Kapila is the proponent of the Sankhya model of creation. The Sankhaya model is composed of 24 principles of creation and is one of the six systems of Indian philosophy.

4 Nyaya is the second system of Indian philosophy. Its proponent is Sage Gautama and propagates knowledge through critical logic and observation.

5 Vaisheseka is the third system of Indian philosophy. Its proponent is Sage Kanada. It specifyies the important aspects of concrete reality. Its theory holds to an atomic theory of existence that claims the entire universe is composed of atoms.

6 Mimamsa is the fourth system of Indian philosophy. Sage Jaimini is its proponent. It emphasizes teachings of the "Vedas". It says the ultimate creator of the universe is God, and God is eternal, timeless, and has a pure existence.

7 Yoga is the fifth philosophy. Sage Patanjali is its proponent. It signifies union of the lower self with the higher self, a union of man and God, a practical guide with 8 limbs.

8 Vedanta is the sixth philosophy. Its proponent is Sage Badarayana. It is formed by two words: "ved" means "knowledge" and "anta" means the "ending". It holds and deals with expansion of consciousness.

by Sage Kapila, the founder of the Sankhya Model of Creation, is the most important among them all. The last three Mimamsa, Yoga, and Vedanta represent the observation of the inner reality to better understand the physical reality. The Sanskrit word "Sankhya" is made up of the words "San" meaning "truth" and "Khya" meaning "to understand to know the truth". Sage Kapila's model of Sankhya-Philosophy considers twenty-four principles in the manifestation of the Universe as we know it.

According to Sankhya Model, all creations need two basic principles. The two essential components for any creation are the male and female energy components. No creation is possible in the absence of either of them. The male energy represents the *Purusha*[9] that is the passive potential energy without its feminine part. The Purusha represents the "pure consciousness" that inhabits the field of senses. He represents choice-less, pure, and passive awareness. Therefore, Purusha is formless, colorless and beyond attributes, transcending duality.

The female energy represents *Prakruti*[10]. She is the reason for creation and has choice, will, and creative potential. It therefore represents the active awareness that yearns to be united with its male counterpart to give birth to creation. Although both Purusha and Prakruti have come together in creation, it is the Prakruti's innate desire that initiated the creation process. Therefore all creation comes from the womb of Prakruti, earning it the right to be called the "Divine Mother". Although matter cannot exist without energy, however energy can exist without matter. The Prakruti cannot exist without the Purusha but Purusha can be without Prakruti.

The union of Purusha and Prakruti gave birth to the first expression of creation: the Cosmic Intelligence. This intelligence pervades each cell. All body processes – be it inside cells or outside of cells or between the cells – are the basis of all communication. This is the flow of intelligence

---

9 Purusha comes from "pur" meaning "city" and "sheta" meaning "dwelling". Purusha is pure consciousness that exists and dwells in city of senses. It is the ultimate truth, ultimate healing power, and ultimate enlightenment.

10 Prakruti is the primordial will. It is primordial matter with creative potential with form, colour, and attributes in the field of action. It is responsible for creation. It is the "Divine Mother".

that is the life force. Have you ever wondered how a single cell becomes a full-grown baby? It is accredited to this innate intelligence. This innate intelligence exists in each molecule of existence. The principle of cause and effect is at the foundation of the theory of creation.

When Prakruti became conscious of the consciousness itself, it created the first expression of cosmic intelligence that is denoted by the *Mahad*.[11] When Mahad became personal, it became an individual intelligence known as the "Buddhi". The identification brings the "I-ness", which gave birth to the *Ahamkara,*[12] or the "Ego". Now the cosmic is an individual. Even though we are in this confined body, we also have the Purusha element in us. It is not easily conceived by us, but regardless it is there. The possibility to attain its awareness is innate in all of us regardless of our limitations. It is accessible to us through us willingly choosing to explore it.

The individual consciousness has three qualities: the pure form is Sattva,the active form (movement) is Rajas, and the inert form (dull and confusion) is Tamas. These are the three qualities (the Gunas) that are laced in all matter and which affect both our body and mind. Be careful not to confuse the inactivity of Purusha with the inactivity of Tamas. In the Purusha form, it is pure consciousness flowing with awareness in an impersonal way, while the inertia in Tamas is devoid of awareness and, therefore, brings sleep, dullness, and confusion. Sattva and Tamas are both static and need momentum from the movement of Rajas to express themselves further.

When the pure consciousness of Sattva interacted with the kinetic energy of Rajas, it gave birth to the five sense faculties, the five motor faculties of action, and the mind (which involves both action and cognition).

The interaction of the kinetic energy of Rajas and the potential energy of Tamas gave birth to the five subtle forms of the great elements called

---

11 Mahad is a supreme creative intelligence. It is born out of a union of Purusha and Prakruti.

12 Ahamkara is the feeling of "I am". It is an individual principle that is centred awareness.

the *Tanmatras:*[13] sound (ether), touch (air), form (fire), taste (water), and smell (earth). There is no sound possible without the presence of the ether element; there is no touch without the air element; there is no form perception without the fire element; there is no taste perception without the water element; and last but not the least, there is no smell perception without the earth element.

The great elements present in nature constantly interact to give birth to the *Tridoshas.*[14] The Tridoshas simply mean the three bio-energies pervading each particle of creation. These bio-energies can be measured and seen both qualitatively and quantitatively in each aspect of creation. "Tri" means "three" and "dosha" means "an entity that can go out of balance".

The Journey of Consciousness into Matter

The union of the male and female energies gave birth to the great elements that constitute and embody all of creation. Nothing in creation exists outside of the scope of these five basic principles. In simple terms, the journey of consciousness to matter is how creation came to be. Therefore a backward journey of matter to pure consciousness is the source of liberation for humankind.

A picture is worth a thousand words, so for your benefit look at the Illustration Flow chart and refer to the twenty-four principles of the creation process as follows.

---

13 Tanmatras comes from the words "tan", meaning "subtle" and "matra", meaning elements. Tanmatras are the subtle elements which are the objects of the five senses: sound, touch, form, taste, and smell. The five senses are hearing, tactile perception, vision, taste, and smell. "Tan" also means "mother" and "matra" means "matter"; together being "the mother of matter". Tanmatras are in the womb of the "Divine Mother". It is the energy that gives rise to the five elements.

14 Tridoshas came from the interplay of the five elements. They are the three bio-energies of vata dosha, pitta dosha, and kapha dosha. They are a functional principle that pervades everyone and everything

Flow Chart 2.1

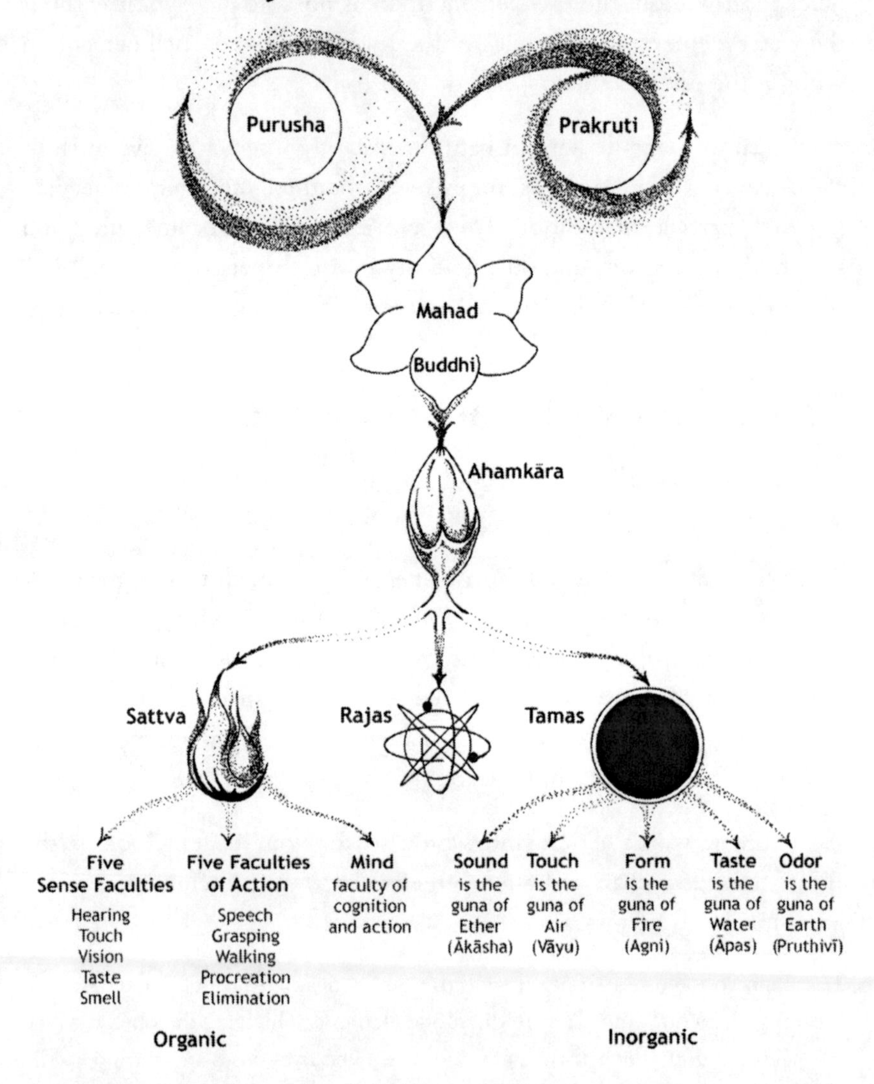

Note: Flowchart 2.1 is credited to the great teacher/Master, Dr. Vasant Lad, whose name is foremost when Ayurveda is the topic of attention. He is a renowned and acclaimed author, artist, and the greatest expounder of Ayurveda in this century. This flow chart is based on work by Dr. Vasant Lad.

Prakruti (Active Component of Creation)
Cosmic Intelligence MAHAD and Individual Intelligence BUDDHI
Ahamkara (Ego)

Three qualities inherent in all creation are the *Sattva*[15] quality, *Rajas*[16] quality, and *Tamas*[17] quality. Sattva and Tamas both are inactive and need the kinetic energy of Rajas to activate and express itself.

Interaction of Sattva and Rajas gave rise to:

Mind: A Faculty of Both Action and Cognition

5 Sense faculties		*5 Motor Organs*
Hearing	↔	Organ of Speech – ears
Touch	↔	Organ of Grasping – hands
Vision	↔	Organ of Walking – eyes
Taste	↔	Organ of Procreation – reproductive organs
Smell	↔	Organ of Elimination – nose

Interaction of Rajas and Tamas gave rise to:

The Five Sensory Perceptions		**The Five- Great Elements**
(The subtle aspect) are the Tanmatras		**(The Gross aspect)**
Sound (Shabda)	↔	Ether (Akasha)
Touch (Sparsha)	↔	Air (Vayu)
Physical Form (Rupa)	↔	Fire (Agni)

15 Sattva; pulsation of cosmic flow caused consciousness to break up into three qualities, Sattva is pure essence of light, right action and spiritual purpose

16 Rajas: is principle of movement, change and excitability

17 Tamas; is inertia, darkness and confusion the three universal qualities has influence over our body and mind

Taste (Rasa)	↔	Water (Jala or Apas)
Odor (Gandha)	↔	Earth (Pruthivi)

The inorganic world is represented in Ayurveda as the five great elements (*panch-bhutas)*[18] of ether (space), air, fire, water, and earth. The great five elements are the micro-building block of all creation – from a blade of grass to the galaxies at large. This is one common entity that binds all animate and inanimate, moving and non-moving, expressions of life as we know on this planet. Nothing exists beyond or out of its scope.

Take a look around and see for yourself: Even if you break down each entity into its molecular components it will still consist of the five elements. What makes a book "a book" and a human "a human" is the proportions in which these five elements align themselves in these entities. What creates the differences is the ratio and vibrations in which the elements exist in any given state of the object in question.

The book you are reading at this instant is made up of the same stuff that you are made up of. Huh? At first glance it's hard to believe, isn't it? But you will see for yourself. The book comes from trees that have all the five elements of nature: roots represent the earth element; sap in the trunks is the water element; the leaves exchanging gas with the environment are the lungs of tree, which is the air element; and the flowers and fruits result from metabolic assimilation of sunlight by the tree, which is the fire element. All of these cannot exist without the space element, which is the subtlest entity of the five elements. Therefore the element of space has all the other elements in its womb.

Now let us look at ourselves. As a person, when we consume the various parts of this plant life, those elements become part and parcel of who we are. The elemental parts of plant life assimilate and nourish our own elements and sustain our existence. The elements configure and are expressed in us at a different vibration and frequency, but still remain essentially the

18 Panch-Bhutas; panch means five, bhutas means elements, panch-bhutas are the five great elements, causative substances are Earth, Water, Fire, Air and Ether

same. Energy is neither created, nor can it be destroyed – although it does change forms.

Our solid parts like bones and muscles are the earth component; our bodily fluids (blood, lymph, sexual fluids) are the water element; the digestive process (considered a metabolic fire) is the fire element, as is sight (which is associated with light); the lungs are the air element; and speech is the expression of the space element. The ratio of the five elements differentiates you from this book in your hand. It is so simple that it is amazing. Today you can safely say I am interconnected to all creation from the grossest to the subtlest.

Table 2.1 Elements vs Sanskrit Name vs Primary Sense Function vs Secondary Motor Function vs Nature

Element	Sanskrit name	Primary Sense Function	Secondary Motor Function	Nature
Ether	Akasha	Sound	Non-resistance	Subtlest
Air	Vayu	Touch	Vibration	Movement
Fire	Tejas	Sight	Heat/ Colour	Transformation
Water	Apas	Taste	Fluidity	Liquid
Earth	Pruthivi	Smell	Solidity	Dense, Grossest

Now we can move on to various functions and the nature of each of these great elements in more detail in the following chapters.

Chapter Three

The Great Elements: The "Panch-Maha Bhutas"

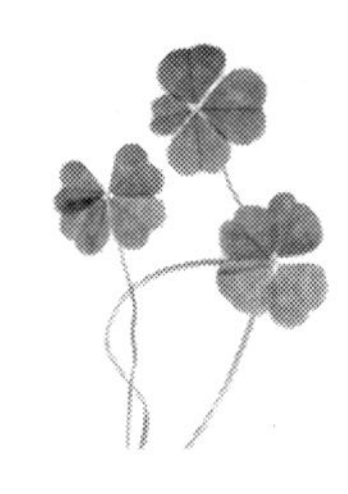

"Five elements – earth, water, fire, air, and ether principles; soul, mind, time, and direction are the nine matter. The substances with manifest consciousness are living, and the substances with un-manifested consciousness are non-living."

—Charaka Samhita, Sutra Section, Ch. 1/48, Longevity

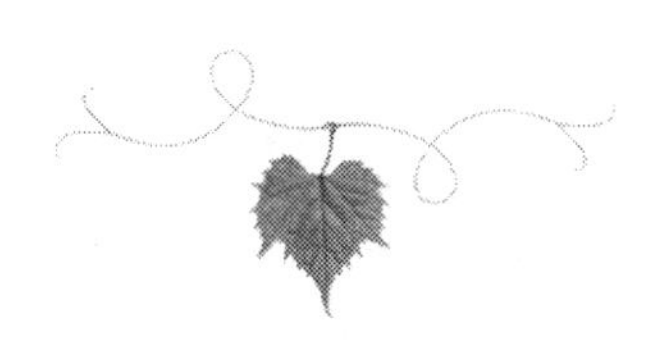

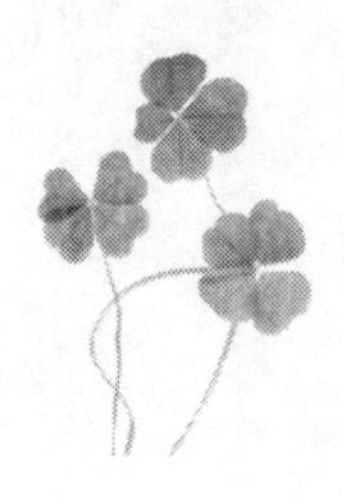

The five elements, thus called the *Panch-Maha-Bhutas,*[19] are the essence of every living cell. They are the building blocks of the whole of existence. Nothing is out of its scope, as mentioned earlier. It is important to know a little bit about each one of these elements as it will be helpful in deeply understanding the basic principles of Ayurveda.

The Ether Element

The first element is ether, or *Akasha* in Sanskrit, meaning all encompassing, omnipresent, omnipotent, and all pervading as it fills any and every empty space. Its qualities are light, clear, soft, subtle, and expanding. Its nature to expand makes it non-resistant, and therefore it provides freedom and love, and deals with the heart of the matter. No music note or verbal talk is possible without the presence of the ether element. It is the space between each note that makes sound possible. Therefore, it is expressed as sound.

It is also the home for all other four elements as this is the subtlest of them all. It carries the rest of them in its womb. Ether was the first expression of consciousness and is the basic need of each cell. Without the space element, nothing could exist. Ether expands to fill all spaces. It is empty and has no resistance; therefore it can make movements of other elements possible by creating space for them. Ether is a pure form of consciousness that manifests itself as nuclear energy.

The Air Element

---

19 Panch-Maha-Bhutas comes from "panch", which means "five" and "Bhutas", which means "elements". Panch-Bhutas are the five great elements, the causative substances of: earth, water, fire, air and ether.

When the same consciousness moves, it becomes the Air element. Therefore, the directional ether element is the air element. The Sanskrit word for air is *Vayu*,[20] and you will see it mentioned as that in other places in the book. Its qualities are movement, dry, light, cold, rough, and subtle. All movements within the body and around our environment are possible due to this element. Its movement is directional; it can move upward, downward, or in a linear or circular manner. This movement quality makes it a vector tool in the diagnostic process.

Air controls the movements of food, nutrition, and waste products into, out, and around the cells, which helps its movement around the body. If upward moving air starts to move downward, it will cause certain changes that are telltale signs of certain conditions. Downward moving air is responsible for excretion, menstruation flow, and the birthing process. Upwards moving air is responsible for movement of the lungs and brain and for stimulating memory. Circular movement occurs around the naval area around the solar plexus. It is responsible for movements in different parts of the small intestine by providing a stimulus for enzyme secretions from the liver and gall bladder for the digestion process. The direction of movement of vayu or air shows its affinity for specific organs and areas of the body. If specific vayu changes from its normal direction, it is bound to cause dysfunctional changes of specific organs. It manifests itself as electrical energy and is represented by the sense of touch.

---

20 Vayu means air and is used as a synonym for vata. There are five main vayus, each named according to its direction. Prana vayu is present in the head and moves downward and inward. Udana vayu is located in the diaphragm and moves upward through the lungs, bronchi, trachea and throat; Udana vayu governs the movement of the diaphragm helping in the process of exhalation hence it is responsible for speech and expression, it is an upward moving vayu. Samana vayu is present in the small intestine and navel and is responsible for creating hunger. Apana vayu is in the pelvic region, cecum, colon, rectum, and urinary tract. It is also present in a downward movement in the male and female reproductive organs. Vyana vayu is present in the heart and maintains its functions throughout the body through the arterial, venous, and lymphatic systems.

The air element's subtle essence is denoted by *Prana,*[21] or "Chi" as in Chinese Tradition. Therefore, Prana is the pure essence of the air element. As air moves through space, it carries with it what comes in its way, making inter-cellular and intra-cellular exchanges of nutrients and gases possible. It is the transporting element. All gross and subtle movements within the cells are due to the flow of Prana. It includes the involuntary movement of the eyelids, lungs, and heart, and the peristaltic movement of the intestines.

Air is the first thing our lungs breathed when we entered the physical world, and air will be the last thing we will breathe when we exit from this world. Breathing air with awareness adds another dimension to this element, which is deep and cleansing at the cellular levels. That is why Ayurveda's sister science of Yoga utilizes the gift of this element to dive deep into other realms beyond the physical body. It has the quality to purify at cellular levels. The yoga practice of conscious breath is healing through *Pranayama,*[22] meaning regulating breath to cleanse deep layers of our tissues, mind, and consciousness itself.

The Fire Element

The movement of the air element creates friction, and friction creates heat, so our next element is fire. This is how awareness took the form of the fire element. Fire means *Agni.*[23] It represents the energy of transformation. Its innate qualities are heat and light. In absence of light, we

---

21 Prana is the basic essence or principle of the air element. It is denoted by the flow of consciousness from one cell to another cell in the form of intelligence. Therefore, it is a vital force and is essential for all subtle and gross movements, including our heart, respiration, peristalsis, and other involuntary movements.

22 Pranayama comes from the words "prana" meaning "vital force" and "yama" meaning "control". Thus, Pranayama means control of a vital force.

23 Agni is the fire element. It governs all transformation and the process of digestion, absorption, and assimilation (be it food or a thought). The Latin word *ignis* and the English word *ignite* has a common root with the Sanskrit word *Agni*. In the cell, Agni is the centre of awareness, governs its functional activities,

lose our sense of direction. The light of knowledge also has subtle aspects of the fire element. To understand something, we need the fire of desire to know it. The fire element's essence is represented in subtle forms as *Tejas*,[24] which represents the flame of pure intelligence. Without the element of fire, food as well as thoughts cannot be processed. Thus, this element maintains body temperature. All sensory perceptions function in its presence – be it the ears, eyes, tongue, nose, or skin. Fire transmutes heavy energy into a ray of pure light. Fire also symbolizes knowledge, while the absence of it results in ignorance. Fire represents radiant energy and the sense of sight. It regulates understanding, comprehension, and the discriminative intellect.

In physical body, this fire resides centrally in the stomach, small intestine, liver, and spleen. Fire circulates through the body via blood and plasma. Fire in the stomach and small intestine is the *Jathara Agni,'*[25] meaning literally "fire in the stomach". It is the centre seat of fire. Touched by fire, nothing remains in its original form, so it is a transformational force. Thus, it forms the base for metabolism, aiding digestion, absorption, and assimilation processes. Digestive fire is the vital force in the maintenance of health. Poor circulation of blood results in cold extremities. Its dysfunction can lead to various disorders. Thus, it deserves its own special mention and is discussed in detail in the chapter on 'Agni'.

---

neutralizes the metabolic toxins (Aam), and maintains cellular intelligence. In modern context, Agni is symbolized by the "digestive enzymes".

24 Tejas is the burning flame of intelligence. The principle of Tejas embraces both light and heat. The illuminated sun represents this quality and is responsible for solar energy. It is the vital subtle energy involved in digestion and transformation of everything from food to a thought to an experience.

25 Jathara Agni is the central fire, which includes Agni in the stomach and small intestines. It governs the initial digestion and is the gateway to the digestive system. Agni has four varieties: balanced (VPK), irregular (vata), sharp (pitta), and slow (kapha).

The Water Element

Heat condenses to form our next element – water. In Sanskrit, it is called "jala" or "apas". It represents chemical energy due to its ionic constitution. Water occupies 70% of the earth as well as our physical bodies. Being a universal solvent, it is essential for cellular functions. Fire in the stomach is contained in a water medium, as stomach acids are crucial for digestion. This is similar to how coolant water circulates around the radiator fluid of a car to prevent it from over-heating. If stomach acids were not contained in the water element, they would break the barriers of the stomach wall and dissolve it.

Therefore, water is essential for assimilation of bodily functions by maintaining electrolyte balance both in inter-cellular and extra-cellular fluids. The plasma part of blood tissue is 90% water in content. It is the medium through which movement of nutrients and the waste products of the digestion process are possible. It manifests as chemical energy and is represented by the sense of taste.

A body's lymphatic system is predominantly made of the water element, making it essential for immunity. Water represents cooling, cleansing, purifying, and balancing. When you are experiencing anger, a cool glass of water can work to cool off your mind.

Water is attracted to gravity, and therefore, always flows towards it. Thus, it symbolizes a heavy nature and the quality of surrender. Water takes on the quality of the things where it is placed, showing its adaptability. Water from a raging river calmly settles into the shape of any container it is put in. When it is put back into the same raging river, it goes back to flowing with the same passionate rage. This is how it teaches us acceptance and flexibility in subtle realms. Sitting near water, be it a river or an ocean, can calm anyone's mind. Water cools, cleanses, purifies, rejuvenates, and revitalizes.

The Earth Element

Water crystallized to its next form, giving birth to the element of earth. The earth element is the densest of the five elements. In Sanskrit, it is called "Pruthivi" and it forms the solid ground for existence. It absorbs all our impurities and uses them as fertilizer to grow the plant life that nourishes and sustains all of creation. It is said to be the "Mother Nature" for us who provides food and support to all life forms. The power vested in it makes it worthy of our gratitude and love as it provides us a "solid base" and roots us to our roots. It is hard, solid, and dense and represents within the human body all solid structures like bones, cartilage, skin, nails, hair, and teeth. It manifests as mechanical energy and is represented by the sense of smell.

The five elements thus form the bases of the life support system that harmonizes this planet and the whole of existence. They maintain the balance and neutralize the dangers that can interfere with nature's balance. The Five elements are continuously changing to accommodate for the changing seasons and climatic conditions. Ayurveda suggests that we must change accordingly to keep all the elements in balance within. All elements are present in each individual, but may differ in combination and proportions. This brings about a unique constitution in each individual.

When one lives a lifestyle conducive to supporting each element through the day and changing seasons, one can maintain harmony and balance in physical, mental, and spiritual endeavours. An increase of any one can lead to an imbalance that presents the need to make adjustments to bring back homeostasis. For example, when the earth element is in excess, it is bound to produce obesity in the physical body and depression, dullness in the mental constitution and greed attachments in spiritual nature. Excess in the water element will cause edema, tumors, and cysts. Increases in the fire element will bring about fevers, hyperacidity, ulcers, hemorrhoids, skin rashes, psoriasis, and inflammatory conditions. Excess in the air element is bound to cause arthritis, indigestion, anxiety, and fear. Imbalance in the ether element will bring about hearing disorders, Parkinson's, Alzheimer's, vertigo, and epileptic seizures.

These five elements therefore form the basic foundation of Ayurveda. The constant interactions of these five elements form the three bio-energies of *Vata,*[26] *Pitta,*[27] *and Kapha.*[28] The ether and air interactions bring about the Vata dosha, the fire and water interactions form the Pitta dosha, and water and earth interactions form the Kapha dosha. Each elemental nature influences the qualities of each dosha. The three doshas therefore form the tripod base foundation on which Ayurveda stands.

The affinity of the three bio-energies to different parts of the body helps in the diagnostic process. By taking care of the prime sites of the doshas – for example, colon for Vata, small intestine for Pitta, and lungs for Kapha – one can maintain an overall healthy balance. The cleansing of the colon, small intestine, and lungs is the main objective of the Panchkarma [29] therapies.

---

26 Vata is one of the three bio-energies present in the body and in nature. It is formed out of the interactions between the ether and air elements. Its prime function is movement. It is responsible for all movements within, around, and between cells. Thus, the exchange of nutrients and the elimination of waste is due to its presence. The prime site of vata in the body is the colon, but it is also present in skin, hair, the lower abdomen, pelvic girdle, thighs, ears, and bones.

27 Pitta is the second of the three bio-energies present in the body and in nature. It is formed out of the interaction between fire and water elements. Its prime function is transformational; all digestive and assimilation processes are due to this energy. The prime site for Pitta is the small intestine, but it is also present in the blood, eyes, the subcutaneous fat of skin, grey matter in the brain, stomach, sebaceous glands, sweat, liver, spleen, and gallbladder.

28 Kapha is the third of the three bio-energies present in the body and in nature. It is formed out of the interactions between earth and water elements. It is the heaviest of the three. Its prime function is stability and lubrication. It maintains cells' integrity. Its prime site is the lungs, but is also present in the plasma of blood, lymph nodes, mastic tissue, synovial fluid, stomach, pancreas, sinus, mouth, nose, throat, tongue, and white matter of meninges in the brain tissues.

29 The term Panchakarma comes from "panch" meaning "five" and "karma" meaning actions. Five actions to cleanse the body/mind/spirit are vomiting, purgatives or laxatives, medicated enemas, nasya (nasal administration of medicated oils or herbal powders) and purification of the blood.

The first action or process in Panchakarma is therapeutic vomiting, called Emesis (or Vamana), to release congestion in lungs where one is experiencing repeated episodes of cough, cold, congestion, and asthma. It is also indicated for skin diseases, diabetes, asthma, edema, chronic indigestion, lymphatic congestion, chronic sinus problems, and recurring tonsillitis. Emetic therapy of Vamana is therefore cleansing by elimination through the upper pathways.

Second in the series of actions are herbal purgatives (Virechana). These help in cases of allergic rash and skin afflictions. It is also the most viable choice of therapies where excess bile is secreted and accumulated in the gall bladder, liver, and intestines. In purgative or Virechana therapies, cleansing is done by elimination through the lower pathways.

The third action in the series is herbal enemas called the "Basti" therapy. It is used to cleanse and tone the colon via elimination and medication through the lower pathways. Vata is mainly located in colon, bones are also site of Vata hence any medication administered rectally also helps deeper tissue of Asthi-dhatu (the bone tissue). It is the choice of treatment indicated in case of constipation, lower back pains, gout, arthritis, sciatica and nervous disorders.

The fourth process is a nasal administration called "Nasya" therapy. In this, medications are administered through the nasal passages to release excessive congestion in the sinuses, nose, throat, and head. The nose is said to be the doorway to the brain and consciousness. It is the choice of treatment for dryness of the nose, nasal polyps, sinus congestion, migraine headaches, convulsions, hoarseness, and various ear and eye problems. There are various types of Nasya therapy according to the need of the situation – whether cleansing, nutritive, or sedative in nature.

Last in the series is blood-letting therapy (Rakta Moksha). When there are excess toxins in the body, the blood is also toxic. Blood-letting therapies are the most efficient choice of therapy in skin disorders like urticaria, scabies, eczema, acne, leukoderma, chronic rashes or hives that itch, and psoriasis. It is therefore applicable and most effective in cases of liver and spleen enlargement or their dysfunctions. This treatment can only be done by a qualified physician. It is not practised in North America due to the nature of the therapy. The blood is a vital fluid and must be protected at any cost. However, it is still practised in some parts of India with the full Panchakarma protocol by qualified physicians.

The elements are one common entity that occupies our body, mind, and soul, and also the Mother Nature, making us a microcosmic reflection of the macrocosmic universe. We are part and parcel of a grand scheme at play. We are One, finding the truth of this idiom is the search of each individual.

Table 3.1 Panchakarma Therapies vs Actions vs Benefits in Conditions

PANCHAKARMA THERAPIES	ACTIONS	BENEFITS IN CONDITIONS
Vamana	Emesis	Congestion in lungs
Virechana	Purgation	Liver and intestines cleanse
Basti	Herbal enemas	Tone & cleanse colon
Nasya	Nasal therapy	Congestive head and sinus, migraines, etc
Rakta moksha	Blood letting	Blood cleansing, liver and spleen

Chapter Four

The Qualities In Nature And Matter: The "Gunas Attributes"

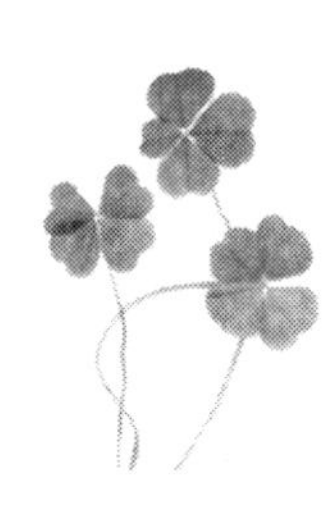

"The soul is the consciousness principle in body. It is our soul that is specifically targeted by Ayurveda because soul or conscious principle is the chief support of life."

—Charaka Samhita, Sutra Section, Ch. 1/46-47, Longevity

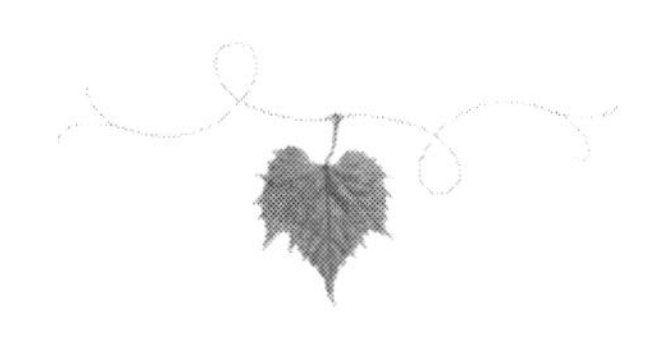

Trigunas: Sattva, Rajas, and Tamas

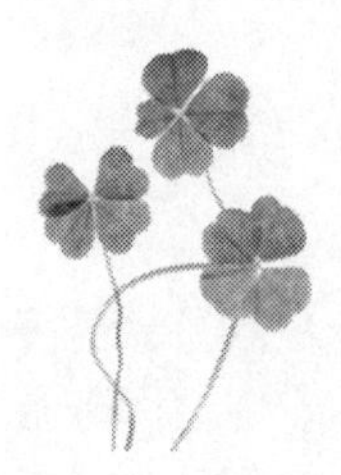

The whole cosmos is connected to our human bodies; each aspect of nature is encoded with certain qualities. These qualitative aspects represent the quality of time, person, place, and objects. Each entity can be represented by any one or two of these qualities, which gives the entity its innate nature. There are three qualities in nature that encompass both our external and internal environments. These qualities are:

Sattva	Pure Intelligence	NUCLEAR ENERGY
Rajas	Action or Movement	CHEMICAL ENERGY
Tamas	Inertia or Darkness	INERT ENERGY

All the three qualities are essential for creation in nature. In the external environment, Sattva represents creative intelligence, Rajas represents active movement, and Tamas represents stagnant inertia. In human beings, Sattva reflects as the supreme discriminative intelligence, Rajas as the "I-ness" or the ego, and Tamas as the darkness represented by innate ignorance.

These qualities are an innate part of everything in nature, and looking deeper, we find that there is a relationship between the five great elements, the three qualities of nature, and the three bio-humours/energies as follows:

Table 4.1 Dosha vs Elements vs Gunas

DOSHA	ELEMENTS	GUNAS
ETHER		SATTVA
VATA	Space + Air elements	SATTVA + RAJAS

DOSHA	ELEMENTS	GUNAS
AIR		RAJAS
FIRE		SATTVA + RAJAS
PITTA	Fire + Water elements	SATTVA + RAJAS
WATER		SATTVA +TAMAS
KAPHA	Water + Earth elements	SATTVA + TAMAS
EARTH		TAMAS

Ten Pairs of Opposites: The Twenty Attributes

Every substance existing in nature can be described by its qualities, which according to Ayurveda, can fit under basic twenty-fold attributes. The twenty attributes exist as ten pairs of opposites. The Sanskrit words for the attributes are included in parenthesis in the table below for your benefit and exploration.

Table 4.2 Ten Pairs of Opposing Attributes Vs Sanskrit Names

Heavy *(Guru)*	Light *(Laghu)*
Slow *(Manda)*	Sharp *(Tikshana)*
Cold *(Shita)*	Hot *(Ushna)*
Oily *(Snigdha)*	Dry *(Ruksha)*
Slimy *(Shlakshna)*	Rough *(Khara)*
Dense *(Sandra)*	Liquid *(Drava)*
Soft *(Mrudu)*	Hard *(Kathina)*
Static stable *(Sthira)*	Mobile *(Chala)*
Subtle *(Sukshma)*	Gross *(Sthula)*
Cloudy *(Avila)*	Clear *(Vishada)*

Upon careful observation, these ten pairs of opposites reveal tremendous insights that can be used in accessing balance and imbalances in an individual. The attributes play an important role in the diagnosis process and the creation of a personalized treatment plan by an Ayurvedic practitioner.

The three bio-energies of Vata, Pitta, and Kapha represent themselves by the nature of their attributes:

Vata tends to be: dry, cold, light, rough, subtle, clear, mobile

Pitta tends to be: hot, sharp, light, mobile, liquid,oily

Kapha tends to be: heavy, slow, dull, oily, dense, slimy, gross, sticky, soft, static, hard

These three bio-energies are further discussed in detail in Chapter 5 on Tridoshas. Here it is briefly mentioned in context of the innate nature of matter and how the elemental constituents of the bio-energies carry the attributes and shape things as we see them. Each attribute has an affinity towards either increasing or decreasing a dosha and affects the strength of an individual's digestive fire (Agni) by increasing it or slowing it down. We will now explore this by taking a look at the pairs of the attributes.

Heavy ~ Light

Here I encourage you to think about which of the five elements are the heavier ones. After careful consideration, you would likely correctly choose the water and earth elements. Now consider which of the three doshas has these elements. It is the kapha dosha. Most heavy qualities therefore will tend to increase kapha and at the same time decrease vata and pitta. Therefore, we can use this quality to decipher that anything heavy will also affect the kapha dosha. The heavy quality lowers the Agni. This knowledge can be applied practically. Following the basic principles of "same increases same" and "opposite balance", one can calm the heavy qualities of kapha imbalances by using light things. Likewise, something heavy can and will balance an increased vata and pitta dosha, owing to their elemental nature of lighter qualities. Pork, beef, lamb, fish, cheeses, sugar, soya beans, and honey are heavy in quality.

The light quality is the opposite of the heavy quality, so it will increase vata and pitta while decreasing kapha, and therefore, increasing Agni. The light quality reduces bulk and dullness while creating clarity and alertness. Most bitter and astringent foods and herbs are light in quality. Mother's milk, goat's milk, cow's milk, rye, black pepper, ghee, mung beans, red lentils, millet, rice, popcorn, sprouts and chicken are the light quality foods.

Therefore in conclusion, the heavy quality will always increase bulk, dullness, and lethargy, while the light nature of things will be helpful in neutralizing the heavy qualities to create a state of balance.

This is how we can use the knowledge in practical, simple ways to create balance when there is imbalance. Now take a moment and look at the other nine pairs and give yourself a little challenge to see if you could apply their benefits in your daily life.

Slow ~ Sharp

The slow quality increases kapha and decreases vata and pitta. The slow quality also decreases Agni. The slow quality causes sluggishness, dullness, relaxation, and calm. Eating ice cream in the dead of winter will slow you down and cause heavy mucus to increase in the body. An elephant is as slow as it is heavy, so most heavy things will cause the slow quality. In foods, these include meat, tofu, and yogurt.

The sharp quality will increase pitta and vata but decrease kapha. The sharp quality will increase Agni. Hot, spicy foods like chillies, cinnamon, saffron, brown meats, ginger, garlic, onion, radishes, horse radish, mustard seeds, and greens are sharp and often improve circulation, understanding, and learning. In excess it can cause ulcers and rashes.

Cold ~ Hot

The cold quality increases vata and kapha but decreases pitta. The cold quality therefore ends up decreasing Agni. Cold causes constriction, anxiety, and fear. It douches Agni, which causes mucus to accumulate. The winter and early spring seasons are cold. Foods like icy cold drinks, cooling spices like coriander and green cardamom, apples, potatoes, melons, peaches, and mint are cold.

The hot quality increases pitta but decreases kapha and calms vata. It is the opposite of cold, and thereby increases Agni and improves circulation, digestion, and assimilation. It melts kapha and helps cleansing. Hot, spicy foods like cayenne pepper, piper longum, bay leaf, fenugreek seeds, brown rice, turmeric, sesame seeds, eggs, and alcohol are hot.

Oily (unctuous) ~ Dry

The oily quality increases pitta and kapha and decreases vata. Oily brings calmness over disturbed vata by relaxing it with its heavy quality. It is moist, emollient, and lubricating, and hence, nourishing. Seed butters and nut butters and oils are source of oily qualities. Love and compassion are unctuous. Foods like chicken, fish, almonds, sunflower seeds, ghee, coconut oil, avocado, and cheeses carry the oily quality. The oily quality will decrease Agni. It is worth noticing that although the avocado is an oily food, it is also a good source of protein and has good HDL cholesterol in its fat. In limited quantity, it can help maintain good balance in cholesterol and triglycerides levels in the body.

The dry quality increases vata and decreases pitta and kapha. It is the opposite of oily and creates dryness and dehydration and can cause constipation and hard, dry stools. It tends to increase the Agni. This quality can cause chocking, constriction, and spasms. It causes dry, rough, and cracked skin, nails, and hair. The feelings of isolation, separation, and loneliness are associated with the dry quality. In foods, rabbit, honey, ginger, black pepper, pumpkin, chickpeas, walnuts, millet, and rye are dry in quality.

Slimy (smooth)~ Rough

The slimy quality increases pitta and kapha and decreases vata. It decreases Agni. Foods like cheeses and oils increase pitta while foods like avocado increase (good) kapha, and therefore, are useful in arthritic conditions. Foods like white rice, okra, chia seeds, flax seeds, banana, ghee, yogurt, avocado, fish, and pork are slimy and smooth in quality.

The rough quality increases vata and decreases pitta and kapha. It increases Agni. It causes dryness, roughness, and constipation. All raw food and beans are astringent and carry the rough quality. Chickpeas, spinach, lettuce, cabbage, cauliflower, celery, okra, ginger powder, and salt are rough in quality.

Dense ~ Liquid

The dense quality increases kapha and decreases vata and pitta. All meats and dairy products are dense. It increases bulk and makes the body compact. It stabilizes vata by grounding it. Denseness decreases Agni. Cheeses, meats, and coconut are dense in quality. Likewise, root vegetables like beets and carrots are all denser than leafy vegetables.

The liquid quality decreases vata and increases pitta and kapha. It decreases Agni. It dissolves and liquefies, increases saliva secretions, and therefore, promotes fluidity. Water and most diluted liquids carry this quality. Increased intake of this quality may cause water retention. Milk and most juicy fruits and vegetables have the liquid quality. Watermelons, young coconut water, grapes, leafy lettuce, celery, cantaloupe, and peaches also have the watery liquid quality.

Soft ~ Hard

The soft quality increases pitta and kapha and decreases vata. This quality decreases Agni. It denotes delicateness, tenderness, and loving kindness. It calms vata conditions, being the opposite of dry and rough. Soft foods like banana, sops, chiku, persimmon, polished white rice, avocado, ghee, and seed and nut oils carry the soft quality.

The hard quality increases vata and decreases pitta, and in excess, increases kapha. It decreases Agni. It increases hardness, rigidity, insensitivity, and callousness. The growth of corns, callouses, and warts on the feet are hard in nature. Cysts, tumors, and lumps in the breasts are an indication of hardness as well. In foods, coconut, almonds, and sesame seeds carry this quality.

Stable ~ Mobile

The static/stable quality increases kapha and decreases vata and pitta. It decreases Agni. It provides stability and support. Sitting still in meditation is static, but carries sattvic quality. The night time is also static and carries the tamasic quality, allowing things to slow down and sleep to invade for a much needed rest. Foods like dry lentils and grains and ghee are stable in nature.

The mobile quality increases vata and pitta and decreases kapha. It increases Agni. It increases agitation and restlessness that affects the body as well as emotions. Increased physical activity, frequently travelling in changing time zones, and jetlag will promote this quality, while sitting quietly promotes the static quality. In foods, sprouts, alcohol, and popcorn carry the mobile quality.

Subtle ~ Gross

The subtle quality increases vata and pitta but decreases kapha. It increases Agni. Any thought that has awareness in it is subtle by nature. The lighter elements of air and ether have the subtle quality and carry acertain lightness in them. Our mind, perceptions, feelings, emotions, and five senses are subtle, while the physical body is gross. Bitter foods are subtle and are needed in small quantities in our diet. It promotes subtle clearing of deeper tissues, making room for flow and happenings. In foods, ghee, honey, and alcohols carry subtle qualities.

The gross quality is the opposite of the subtle quality. It is heavier in quality and increases kapha while decreasing pitta and vata. It decreases Agni. The earth element is the grossest of the five elements, while the water element has both gross and liquid qualities. Our physical body and associated earthy things are gross. In foods, meats, cheeses, and mushrooms carry the gross quality.

Cloudy, Sticky ~ Clear

The cloudy quality decreases vata and pitta, but increases kapha. It decreases Agni. This quality promotes unclearness and confusion and heals broken bones. In foods, black lentils (urd-dal), yogurt, and cheeses carry this cloudy quality.

The clear quality, as its name suggests, increases vata and pitta, but decreases kapha while increasing Agni. The sharp pungent tastes have a clearing quality. Heating pungent honey and ginger melts mucus and is helpful in clearing it. A clear mind and thoughts promote self-awareness, which brings on detachment and isolation. In foods, fresh water and vegetable and fruits juices all carry the clear quality.

Ayurveda propagates the mantra *same increases same while opposite qualities balance*. One can apply this deduction in one's day-to-day lives. Thus, the practical knowledge of five great elements, three bio-energies, three basic qualities of nature, and ten pairs of opposite qualities form the complete overview of Ayurveda in a simple yet effective way.

The universal nature of these essential aspects is timeless. Therefore it can be applied anytime to anything to make its wisdom available. This knowledge can help us live our present day lives while applying its immortal wisdom. Once understood deeply, it can simply unfold its secrets to open aspirants generously. Such is the gracious gift of the ancient times to modern-day human and their ailments. It is the only way the ancient can find its relevance in the present day.

Ayurveda is eternal, and its pure knowledge has survived the passage of time. It continues to adapt itself to the changing times and continues to shower us with its simple and effective wisdom. Often a theory can be rendered useless with changing times, but only eternal truth can last through changing times without losing its efficacy.

Ayurveda's approach has been about prevention and this makes it a timeless treasure in these challenging times. There is no relief in sight to ending chronic diseases using conventional modern medicine. However, Ayurveda comes to the rescue and lives up to its promise of delivering vitality and longevity compassionately to each interested individual.

Each day is divided into the continuous play of these three qualities (*the Gunas*) and the three doshas, which are influenced further by their innate ten pairs of opposing qualities. This principle applies to our twenty-four hour day cycle, life-span cycle, and the seasonal cycles.

The twenty-four hour daily cycle is divided into the three doshas as follows:

6 to 10 a.m./p.m.: denotes kapha times, tamasic by nature, owing to its heavy qualities

10 to 2 a.m./p.m.: denotes pitta times, rajasic by nature, owing to its light, fiery qualities

2 to 6 a.m./p.m.: denotes vata times, sattvic by nature, owing to its subtle light qualities

The time of the day or the night has an affinity toward the specific organs. Thus the timing of when various symptoms appear can tell an Ayurvedic practitioner which organ is being adversely affected. This is an important tool in the diagnosis and prognosis process in Ayurveda.

Life-span enumeration is also associated with the rhythm of nature:

Infancy to 12 years is the kapha age and is tamasic in quality: This makes infants and children carefree and happy-go-lucky. They are prone to most congestive disorders.

13 to 50 years (time for work and to earn one's livelihood) is the pitta age and is Rajasic in quality: Studies, marriage, career, and establishing oneself happens during this phase of life. In this stage of life, one is prone to pitta-genic disorders affecting the liver and spleen that can cause conditions like psoriasis, eczema, high cholesterol, diabetes, etc.

50+ years (the golden age) is the Vata age and is Sattvic in quality: It is time for rest and one naturally moves towards introspection in this stage of life. One is prone to most vata-genic disorders in this phase, like arthritis, osteoporosis, Alzheimer's, emphysema, bronchitis, asthma, Parkinson's, senility, etc.

Seasonal cycles are also governed by these qualities as follows:

Winter ~ early spring: kapha seasons

Summer ~ early autumn: pitta seasons

Fall ~ early winter: vata seasons

There is a constant applicability that can be applied to maintain a state of balance once we know what time of day, what age, and what seasonal cycle is involved to make best use of the wisdom that Ayurveda has to offer.

Chapter Five

The Tridoshas: The Tripod of Ayurveda – "You are Unique" Says Ayurveda

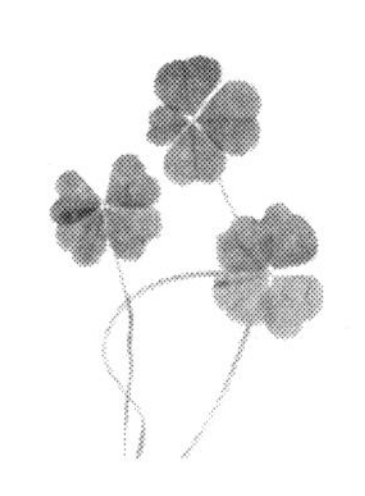

"The tri-fold knowledge of cause (hetu: aetiology), diagnosis (ling: signs to know) and therapeutic modalities (aushadh), with respect to healthy and diseased persons, are of the greatest significance. The knowledge of trisutra (tripod of Ayurveda) is eternal (shashuat) and beneficial (punyam), and is known (cognized) by Brahma himself."

—Charaka Sutrasthanam

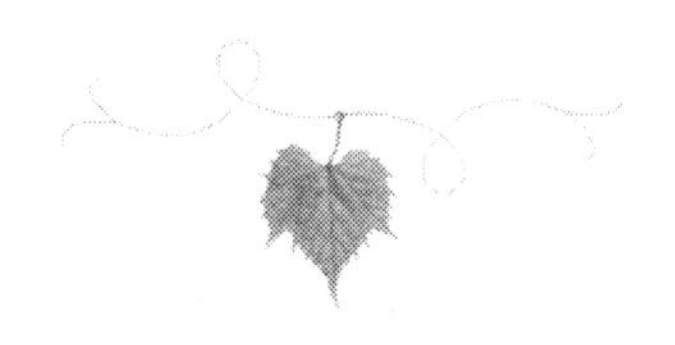

"You Are Unique" Says Ayurveda

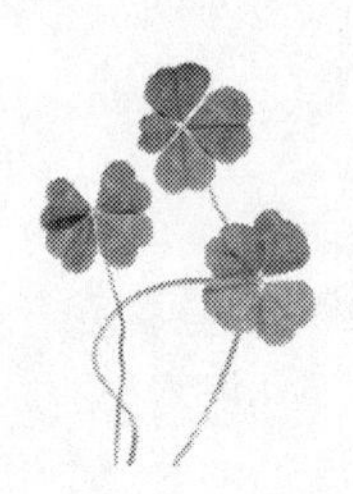

Owing to this ancient wisdom, we are all unique individuals. The unique way in which the tridoshas assimilate in our physical, mental, and cosmic reality leaves its one-of-a kind blueprint just as in conventional medicine DNA constitutes one's individual imprint. Similarly in Ayurveda, the uniqueness lies in an individual's personal constitution.

Personal constitution is a conceptual reality that remains unchanged throughout one's life time. This is unlike modern medicine in which individuals are although identified by DNA mapping, but are not further segregated as one person from another person.

Ayurveda suggests that an individual's constitution is personal and unique. No two individuals are considered the same in Ayurveda, even though they may have the same constitution. Within the same constitution, two people can have different attributes of the dosha display itself.

For example, in a vata prime dosha individual one might be drier and another person might be colder. Hence, the attributes' innate qualities differentiate these two people even though their prime dosha is the same. This is a special feature of Ayurveda and enables one to deeply look at each manifestation of existing doshas. This feature makes it an authentic individualized holistic health care system in the world.

In each moment, the elements collaborate in one's body to determine his or her present state of health. This denotes the individual's temporary imbalances.

An Ayurvedic practitioner uses this knowledge of the two bio-metres of genetic dispositions (constitution) and present state of health (imbalances), to bring about a state of balance in an individual and a state of health and well-being. The concept of personal constitution (*Prakruti)*[30] and the

30 The constitution is called Prakruti. In Sanskrit, this term simply means the very nature. It is the primordial matter; the first expression of creation. It denotes

present state of imbalance (Vikruti)[31] is a unique feature of Ayurveda. Ayurveda applies different modalities at its disposal – be it lifestyle management, nutritional recommendations, herbal supplementation, and/or therapeutics – to bring back an individual to his or her balanced constitution. Once the individual returns near to his/her balanced constitution, health prevails. To achieve this constitutional balance is the objective of an Ayurvedic consultation.

Interplay of Five Great Elements: The Tridoshas

The concept of triple bio-energies, the Tridoshas, is the backbone of Ayurvedic principles. This term comes from "tri"", meaning three, and "dosha", referring to the entity that can go out of whack. The interplay of the basic five elements gave birth to the principle of Tridosha.

Space and the air elements' interactions gave rise to the **Vata dosha.**

Fire and the water elements' interactions gave rise to the **Pitta dosha.**

Earth and the water elements' interactions gave rise to the **Kapha dosha.**

Vata, Pitta, and Kapha form the tripod base on which this ancient wisdom of Ayurveda rests.

Space (or the ether) element + air element = Vata dosha (**together form the movement principle)**

---

how the basic five elements express themselves in an individual. Prakruti is determined at the time of conception and remains unaltered throughout one's life.

31 Vikruti is the combination of elements, however, it is continuously changing moment to moment. It reflects changes in the seasons, times of day, and stages of life to form physical and pathological changes in body, mind, and spirit alike. Bringing Vikruti to match an individual's Prakruti is how a Ayurvedic practitioner brings about balance and healing.

Fire element + water element = Pitta dosha (**together form the metabolic transformation principle)**

Earth element + water element = Kapha Dosha **(together form the cohesive and lubrication principle)**

All the three bio-energies are present in everything and everyone at all times. Generally speaking, there is no 'Vata' without movement, there is no 'Pitta' without transformation and lastly there is no Kapha without cohesiveness. All three entities govern each function at cellular, tissue, organ, and organism levels.

Take a single cell's activity and observe it closely: without the vata principle, there would be no exchange of fluids or gases among cells owing to its movement quality within and around cells. And without pitta, the digestion and assimilation of energy at cellular level would not occur. Likewise, without kapha, the integrity of the cellular membrane itself would cease to exist. In essence, the three bio-energies therefore keep the cells alive and functional through times immortal. Understanding this basic principle is of utmost importance before we can move forward.

Individual Qualities of Each Dosha

The elements of which a dosha is made up of influences the characteristics of that dosha. Now we can apply the knowledge of the attributes of the "ten pairs of gunas" to further deepen our understanding of the characteristics of the three doshas. Each elemental component effects and shows its face in the physical, mental, and spiritual aspects of the total being.

Once we understand the mechanics of each dosha, we can truly apply the knowledge to understand how and why each individual behaves, reacts, and responds to different situations and circumstances. This can open a new vista to look at each individual with the eyes of compassion. We cannot escape the effects doshas have on our physique, mental makeup, and spiritual inclinations that are the realities of our doshas.

Each dosha is under the influence of its constituent elemental qualities, and each quality gives it its flavour and represents those qualities. There are seven basic types of constitutions: V, P, K, VP, PK, VK (or PV, KP, KV), and VPK, although single dosha constitutions are rare, they do exist. The most common are the dual-dosha constitutions. And the rarest of them all is the triple dosha constitution ofVPK, where the three doshas exist in equal proportions.

Once you complete the chart "finding your constitution" in Appendix IV, add the scores at the bottom of each dosha. For example, if your V-score is 50, P score is 40, and K-score is 10, your constitution will be written as V3P2K1, meaning your prime dosha is vata, your secondary dosha is pitta, and third dosha is kapha. This does not makeup for a proper evaluation by an Ayurvedic Practitioner.

Discussing each type of constitution is beyond the scope of this book and neither is it the intent. However, we shall examine the individual nature of each dosha. Two people with the same dosha constitution can be different owing to the subtle qualities of the ten pairs of opposites. For example, vata qualities are clear, light, mobile, dry, cold, rough, astringent and brownish-black. Any two vata-predominant constitution individual could be different in nature owing to how one can be more dry than cold or rough. This explains why no two individuals of the same constitution can be same. This gives Ayurveda its ability to treat each person as a unique individual rather than compiling everyone in one group. There is no other like you, and thus, Ayurveda is a holistic personalized preventive health-care modality.

Upon a closer look at the physical, mental, and spiritual makeup of each dosha constitution, you might find yourself relating to more than one type of dosha constitution. This simply means you have a dual-doshic constitution. Or if you find yourself in each dosha equally, you have a triple- doshic constitution. For fun, there is a constitution evaluation chart given in appendix IV at the back of this book. It is suggested you fill this chart out at different times throughout your life to help you to analyze yourself. You will see for yourself, how the changing seasons and changing stages of your lives your present state changes. However constitutionally, you remain essentially the same.

Characteristics of a Vata Constitution Individual

The Sanskrit term vata is derived from the verb "vah" meaning a vehicle that moves and carries. Vata is the mobility and movement principle that applies to all activities in the body – be it the movement of food through the intestines or movement of thoughts in the mind.

The elements of air and ether influence vata individuals at each stage of their lives. Owing to vata's elemental qualities, they display as dry, light, cold, rough, subtle, mobile (erratic), clear, astringent, and brownish-black. Vata individuals have these attributes influencing their physical body characteristics, mental makeup, and emotional/spiritual qualities.

Dry attributes make them have dry hair, skin, lips, tongue, and colon, which can tend towards constipation, having a hoarse voice, and crackling joints. Physically, the light quality tends to give them a light bone frame with thin muscles and large protruding teeth. They tend to be underweight and either too small or too tall in body height. Sleep is scanty for them. They have small, recessed dry eyes. Their irregular and erratic nature follows in their appetites, thirst, digestion and mal-absorption. They tend to have issues with their health throughout their lives, and shy away from having children (tending to have few or none).

They have cold hands and feet due to poor circulation and are always trying to feel warm.

The mobile quality is visible in their fast-paced life. They tend to be fast talking and walking and do many things at one time, making them restless individual with restless eyes. They love constant change and get bored with the "same old same", making them move place to place and even change furniture in a room just to keep themselves from getting bored.

They love to travel as a variety of new things fascinate them. They are known to experience mood swings, shaky faith, and scattered mindset.

But clear qualities enable them to be clairvoyant, quick to learn, and quick to forget. They can experience clear, empty minds along with bouts of void and loneliness. Vata individuals are prone to anxiety and nervousness disorders.

They tend to have dry scratchy throats and be prone to hiccups and burping. They love warm, oily foods with sweet, sour, and/or salty tastes. Pungent, astringent, and bitter tastes tend to aggravate them. They tend to have dark complexions, dark eyes, dark hair colour, and a dark coated tongue. For a vata pacifying diet, please refer to Appendix I at back of the book.

Characteristics of a Pitta Constitution Individual

Pitta comes from the Sanskrit word "tap", meaning to heat and to display self-discipline. Pitta is influenced by its elemental constituents of fire and water. It is associated with all metabolic activities in and around the body, mind, and spiritual endeavours. The quality of transformation is the core essence of the pitta dosha.

The fire element is literally contained in the water element and represented by the central digestive fire in the stomach as stomach digestive enzymes. The stomach enzymes contain the amino acids crucial for all metabolic activities. The neurotransmitters in the brain, which are responsible for comprehension and thinking processes, are nothing but fire contained in water. It is the presence of the water element in a pitta dosha that prevents the enzymes from eating away its own protective mucus lining of the stomach walls.

Pitta dosha is influenced by its elements and reflects in these individuals with qualities like hot, sharp, light, liquid, spreading, oily, sour, pungent, bitter, fleshy, smelly, and the colours red and yellow.

Due to fiery hot attributes, pitta individuals are blessed with a good digestive fire associated with a strong appetite and a hot body temperature that makes them shy away from hot temperate climates. They are equally thirsty for knowledge and are capable of deep understanding.

Pitta individuals tend to grow grey early and have a receding hairline or even baldness. They have soft, brown, straight hair on their body and face.

The sharp quality gives them sharp teeth, sharp piercing eyes, a pointed nose, and tapering chin. They may even have a heart-shaped face. They usually have good absorption complementing their strong digestion. They are gifted with a sharp memory and sound understanding. Due to their sharp intellect and thirst for knowledge, they do well in various academic fields and become renowned in noble professions. But they are quick-tempered and get irritated easily. They have a light to medium body frame. They tend to have radiant, shiny skin and bright expressive eyes. They tend to have loose bowels; constipation is a word that does not exist in their vocabulary. They have soft and delicate muscles. Urine is excessive as is thirst and sweat in hot summer climates especially.

Owing to pitta's spreading mobile quality, they are easy to break into a rash and acne and are prone to inflammatory conditions. They are conscious of their vanity and enjoy name and fame. They usually make great orators and leaders. They tend to have oily skin and hair. They have tapering, strong, radiant artistic nails.

They are sensitive to hot, spicy and fried foods. Excessive consumption of these foods can cause, vomiting, nausea, and migraine headaches. They are quick to suffer from sour stomachs and acidic pH, and have sensitive teeth due to excessive salivation. Heartburn and acid indigestion are common to pitta individuals. They are quick to anger and have strong feeling of hate if things do not go their way. They are quick to judge and criticize and settle for nothing but perfection in everything they take on. They also tend to be impatient in situations where things go slower than anticipated.

They may have a bitter taste in their mouth upon waking when in state of imbalance, which can make them cynical. Due to strong, open sweat glands, they tend to have strong body odours. They can have a fetid smell under their armpits, in their mouth, and the soles of their feet (indicated by smelly socks). They have red, flushed skin, eyes, cheeks, and nose.

Red is fire colour and can aggravate them. They sometimes tend to have yellow eyes, skin, urine, and feces. A strong tendency towards liver dysfunctions can lead to jaundice due to an over production of bile (a pitta component). The yellow colour is indicative of increased pitta, whereas a pale yellow is normal pitta. A dark yellow is pitta with Aam (metabolic toxins).

Bitter, astringent, and sweet tastes are soothing to pitta while pungent, sour, and salty are aggravating tastes. For a pitta pacifying diet, please refer to Appendix II at the back of this book.

Characteristics of a Kapha Constitution Individual

Kapha comes from two Sanskrit root words: "ka", meaning "water", and "pha", meaning "to flourish". Thus, it literally means "that which flourishes with water". Kapha dosha is made up of the elements of earth and water. Both these elements are gross, heavy, and stable, giving kapha individuals their cohesive and lubricating qualities. Both these elements have a strong affinity for gravity, and therefore, these individuals are gifted with a stable, strong grounding in all three aspects (physical, mental, and spiritual). Kapha's nature gives cell walls their structural integrity. It gives lubrication to joints and shape and weight to the body.

Elemental influences of earth and water give these individual qualities of heavy, slow, cool, oily, liquid, dense, soft, static, cloudy, sticky, hard, and gross nature.

The heavy quality is evident in heavy bones and a broad body frame. They tend to be over-weight. They are grounded individuals with a strong, stable faith.

Slow and dull qualities make them slow in walking, talking, digestion, and metabolism.

They have cool, clammy skin, but steady appetites and thirst with slow metabolism and digestion. This makes them prone to repeated outbreaks of cold, congestion, and cough.

The lubricating quality of the water element gives this constitution well-nourished, oily skin and hair. Even their bowel tends to be well-formed, tubular, and somewhat heavy and oily in nature. They are graced with well-lubricated, unctuous joints and organs.

They have smooth internal organs, as well as smooth skin and calm and gentle minds.

The dense quality of their elements gives them thick hair and makes them overweight due to a dense pad of adipose fat, which makes them thick skinned with firm, rounded bodies and compact, condensed tissues.

Softness and pleasing manners are innate qualities of these individuals. They tend to have soft, loving eyes and a caring, loving, kind, forgiving, and compassionate nature.

The static nature of their elements make them dull, easygoing individuals, who love to do nothing but sit, eat, and sleep leisurely. They tend to save money easily, spending seldomly, and then only for sweet treats.

The sticky quality makes them viscous and compact, with firm joints and muscles tissues. They like to hug and are deeply attached to their loved ones. In an imbalanced state, they tend to be greedy and attached.

Owing to its cloudy nature, they are slow to move and learn, but their retaining power is strong.

Hardness gives them a firm muscle structure and a good stable strength that matches their equally rigid attitudes.

The gross quality makes them prone to obesity and congestive disorders. It makes it hard for them to shed excess weight.

Sweet attributes denoted by their anabolic nature can stimulate sperm formation and increase and improve the quality of semen. However, its abnormal functioning may lead to unhealthy cravings for excess sweets.

Salty attributes help with digestion and in maintaining the osmotic condition in the body. While an imbalance in the salty taste can lead to a craving for salt, and hence, water retention in these individuals.

Kapha is represented by a white colour, pale complexion, white mucus, and a white, thick coating on the tongue due to kapha with Aam (the metabolic toxins in the gastro-intestinal tract).

Sweet, salty, and sour are aggravating to Kapha individuals, while the heating and light qualities of pungent, astringent, and bitter tastes are soothing and balancing to them.

Kapha doshas is the strongest of the three doshas. In the balanced state, these individuals are graced with a warm, caring, loving, compassionate, and forgiving personality. While in the imbalanced state, they tend to be attached, possessive, and lazy.

As you read through the individual characteristics, you will see yourself reflected in certain places, as all three doshas are in all of us at all times.

Keep in mind, an individual is rarely just one dosha and usually dual or triple doshic. As you familiarize yourself with the innate nature of each dosha, you will be more apt to see your own native traits in both the balanced and imbalanced state.

This is a viable tool to practice true understanding within yourself and in relationships. It is your doshas that makes you who you are at any given point and time in your life. Understanding their true nature will help you to better understand yourself. Further, it enables you to better understand others around you – be it your parents, siblings, partner, children, friends, and/or co-workers. Better understanding can lead to a better relationship with self and others.

Practical aspects of knowing your true nature helps you in to find that right job, career, and compatible life partner. Living conducive to your doshas will make the journey of life not only more interesting but equally rewarding.

Before we move forward, a brief mention of the digestive fire (Agni) is needed at this juncture. Healthy fire is an indicator of sound health. According to the Ayurveda doctrine: *You are as healthy as your fire* (meaning the digestive fire).

Chapter Six

The Digestive Fires: The Concept of "Agni"

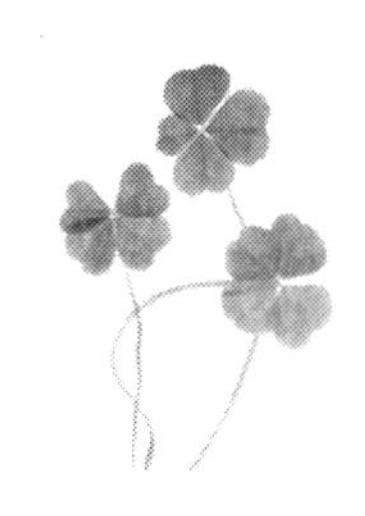

"One who is established in Self, who has balanced doshas, balanced Agni, properly formed dhatus, proper elimination of malas, well functioning bodily processes, and whose mind, soul, and senses are full of bliss, is called a healthy person."

—Sushruta Samhita, 15.38

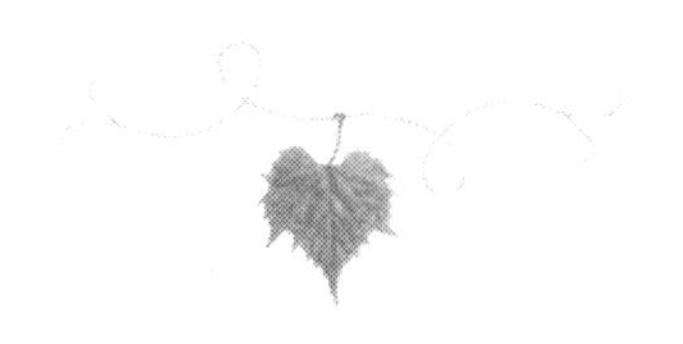

What is "Agni"?[32]
The Digestive Enzymes

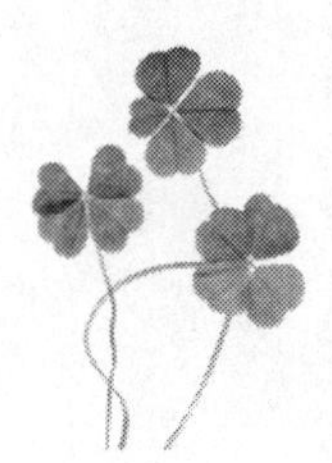

The digestive fire represents the fire element in the body. It governs all transformational functions of the body. Its functions entail digestion, absorption, and assimilation through transformation of food energy (a gross energy) to a subtle energy that governs the functioning of the major functions of all systems in the body.

Along with the tridoshas, the next important factor to consider in any Ayurvedic understanding is the functional integrity of a person's digestive fire. Agni is a fire that transforms food, as well as thoughts, through digestion, assimilation, and absorption. It converts food into heat, energy, vitality, and immunity. It encompasses all three levels (the physical, mental, and spiritual dimensions), making it a holistic complete package.

Agni is the prime source of life, and in its absence, no life is possible. Its external counterpart in nature is represented by the sun. We all know that without the sun there is no life possible on this planet. The same holds true of the human body, internally. Optimal functioning of this life force determines the real age of a person. A slow Agni will slow down the body functioning, as a over-active Agni will eat away and waste the body's own tissues. Thus the Agni can slow or accelerate the aging process. Similarly, a healthy Agni means a healthy immune system, and therefore, a healthy

32 Agni is the digestive fire. In modern context it represents the various digestive enzymes; There are 40 main types of Agnis or enzymes present in various organs in the body, namely stomach, pancreas, choroid plexuses, thyroid, thymus, and 5 in the liver as liver enzymes. There are seven dhatu agnis one for each of the seven dhatus, digestive enzymes are also present in the cell membrane and the cell nucleus,5 enzymes representing the five sense organs, 15 dosha agnis (5 for each one of the 5 subdoshas of the three dosha of VPK) and three malas agnis(For three waste products) namely; sweat, urine and feces.Agnis therefore represent all of the metabolic functions in the body

body, sound mind, and kindled spirit. This is the way a healthy Agni can and does help in the retardation of the aging process. In Ayurveda, there is a famous quote: *A person is as old as his or her Agni.* A young person with a sluggish Agni will look a lot older than an elderly person with a robust Agni.

Did you ever observe that when you are feeling under the weather, you feel cold and have the shivers and a lack of appetite? Did you ever wonder why? It is all due to a sluggish digestive fire. This is the body's own intelligence at work. This is its way of throwing out of the excessive toxins that collect over time and burden and hinder the proper functioning of the digestive fire. Taking warm, soft, and simple foods will rekindle the digestive fire. Fasting is the best way to give an over-burdened body a much-needed relief. Good hunger also means a good digestive fire. Thus, the return of an appetite is considered a sign of regaining back the proper functioning of this transformational force. In death, the body turns cold. Why? Because, when the Agni is extinguished, it stops all body functions.

Functioning of the digestive fire also governs the maturation and maintenance of all seven body tissues. Proper functioning leads to proper production of the rest of the body tissues, and improper functioning produces immature body tissues that are clogged with metabolic waste. Ayurveda calls this metabolic toxic waste Aam. Wherever this toxic metabolic waste lodges, it hinders the functioning of that organ or body tissue. The next time you get sick, do not fret about it. Your body's own intelligence is trying to bring back a balance. It manages to discourage you from continuously indulging in unhealthy food habits. Take the clue to refrain from eating, so your body can regain its own vigour and appetite on its own.

Metabolic waste clouds the cellular intelligence and starts a domino effect at various sites creating a dis-ease. Therefore Agni in the body is represented by the body temperature, digestive enzymes, amino acids, and all metabolic functions.

Fruits and vegetables are loaded with sun energy trapped inside, making the nutrition readily bio-available after consumption. Therefore, most fruits and some vegetable can be consumed raw. With minimum processing, their nutrient content can nourish our being. So it is reasonable to say that without Agni, no digestion is possible.

A proper and robust digestive fire can make up for the short-term negligence of unhealthy food habits and an improper life-style. But an improper digestive fire – whether too slow, fast, or somewhat in between – can render the most healthy food habits and good life-style completely useless. Therefore, foremost attention must be given to one's digestive abilities. Healthy Agni can clear the body of toxic waste faster, compared to a weak Agni in an individual. Therefore, keeping the Agni in order is one of the most beneficial gifts this ancient wisdom has to offer.

The use of many Agni-igniting herbs is recommended in Ayurveda. One of the most common of such herbs is fresh ginger root. If I had to pick one herb that is a solution to all ailments, it would be this herb. Its health benefits and applications are countless. Regardless of one's constitution, one can benefit from its healing abilities. Wisdom lies in its innate qualities and the quantity to be consumed for each constitution. For example, a vata and kapha individual can benefit in larger doses without causing any aggravation. A pitta dosha also can tolerate this amazing herb owing to its unexplainable "special effect", but with some caution. It will be discussed in detail under the chapter of 'The Tastes" later. (Please refer to Chapter # 7 on tastes to clarify the term "special effect" in certain food and herbs).

Proper Agni functions can encourage the various body functions to perform at their optimal best. A robust Agni reduces the production of metabolic toxins produced by improper digestion. The damage caused at the gastrointestinal level gets multiplied into malformation of the deeper tissues like Rasa (plasma), Rakta (blood), Mamsa (muscle), Meda (adipose fat), Asthi (bone), Majja (bone marrow and nerve), Shukra (the male reproductive tissue), and Artava (female reproductive tissue). These body tissues are called *Dhatus* [33]in Sanskrit.

---

33 Dhatus comes from the Sanskrit word "dha", which means "holding, containing, and causing". Dhatu means tissues that hold the organ together. It is the constructing and cementing material of the body. There are seven dhatus: Rasa (plasma), Rakta (blood), Mamsa (muscle), Meda (adipose fat), Asthi (bone

Types of Agni – It's Importance for Total Well-being

Table 6.1 Bodily Tissue Vs Corresponding Dhatus

BODY TISSUE NAMES	DHATUS NAME
PLASMA	RASA
BLOOD	RAKTA
MUSCLE	MAMSA
ADIPOSE FAT	MEDA
BONE	ASTHI
BONE MARROW AND NERVES	MAJJA
REPRODUCTIVE TISSUE SEMEN AND OVUM	SHUKRA MALE AND ARTAVA FEMALE

The main digestive Agni resides in the stomach, liver, and pancreas. The digestive enzymes secreted by these organs rule this process of body tissue formations. Healthy Agni can either promote healthy tissues or slow its process down due to sluggish digestive fire. The malfunctioning of the individual Dhatu Agnis present inside each Dhatu can produce immature body tissues, thereby creating imbalances in an individual. The immature body tissues are unstable and form poor quality of mature body tissues.

The whole process of health depends on the health of our body tissue. Poor Agni causes poor tissue formation, leading to various present-day health concerns. Our ancestors ate simple, pure foods and lead simple lives. But today, modern humans have come far from their original simplicity.

---

tissue), Majja (bone marrow), Shukra (semen), and Artava (ovum). All tissues have a precursor state, mature state, superior state, and inferior state, and inferior and superior by-products. Health in the precursor state produces healthy mature tissues and influences its volume and quality both.

Today modern humans have poor eating habits and a sedentary life-style. Therefore, modern humans face epidemics like obesity, diabetes, cardiac diseases, cancer, brain disorders and various neurological nervous disorders. The list is endless, but on careful observation, the answer is simple.

It requires a responsible commitment on a personal level to respect the old traditions and revisit them to bring about alignment to nature. It is a matter of personal choice and responsibility to follow through with these choices.

Normal functioning of the digestive fire provides us with digestion of food along with the digestion of sensory perceptions. The five senses are the subtle forms of the five great elements. The outcome of sensory digestion is knowledge and cognition. Improper digestion of food causes improper sensory perceptions that can lead to indigestion, constipation, and diarrhea, as well as confusion, irritability, and depression due to the suppression of emotions.

All body functions can be divided into two types: *anabolic*[34] and *catabolic.*[35] When there is an increase in anabolic activity, growth results. While increased catabolic activity causes deterioration or emaciation. This is how a robust Agni acts as a buffer to maintain a balance between the anabolic and catabolic activities within the body. A healthy person represents a healthy Agni and this shows itself as joy, contentment, happiness, and adaptability to life's challenges. Unhealthy Agni causes diseases, while healthy Agni gifts us with wholesome life choices in spite of adverse circumstances.

Robust Agni promotes health of *doshas, dhatus, malas,*[36] senses, mind and consciousness. This creates qualities like a healthy sense of self, joy of life, trust in the unknown, love for all, and harmony in each aspect of life.

---

34 Anabolic means those body functions that increase mass and volume, hence promoting tissue production.

35 Catabolic means those body functions that decrease mass and volume, causing the wasting of tissues leading to emaciation.

36 Malas are the body's post-digestion waste products. They are feces, urine, and sweat.

This single entity is a gift to us from Mother Nature. We must thrive to guard and protect this gift through healthy, fresh food options and a balanced life-style.

Always protect your Agni by eating only foods that can enhance each other when combining them. If two or more foods that have different tastes, energies, and post-digestive effects are combined, it can over-burden your Agni. But the same foods, when consumed separately, can have stimulating effects on Agni by easily digesting and promoting burning of accumulated body toxins (Aam). Foods are further discussed in detail in Chapter # 7. Please also refer to the food-combining table in Appendix V at the end of this book.

Chapter Seven

The Tastes: Precursor to a Balanced Diet

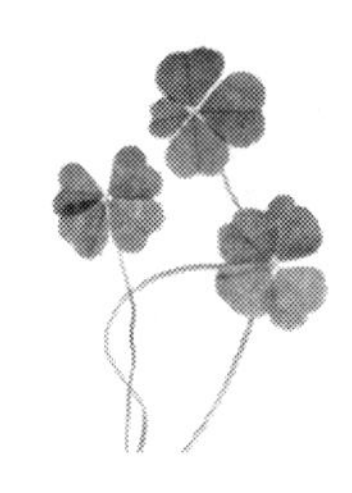

"The water falling from the sky has qualities of moon. They are soft, cool, and without any taste. When this water mixes with the elements located on the earth, Viz, plants, animals, etc, they attain different rasas."

—Charaka Samhita

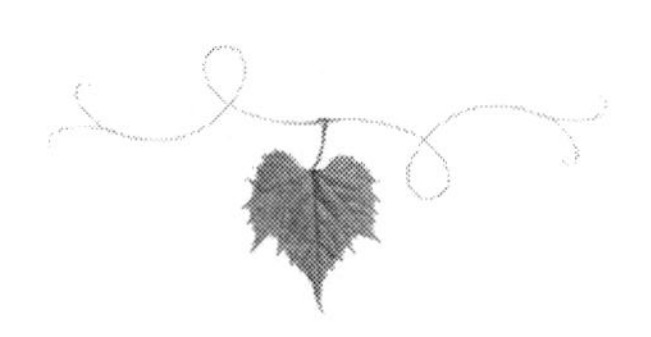

Tastes – the Rasa[37]

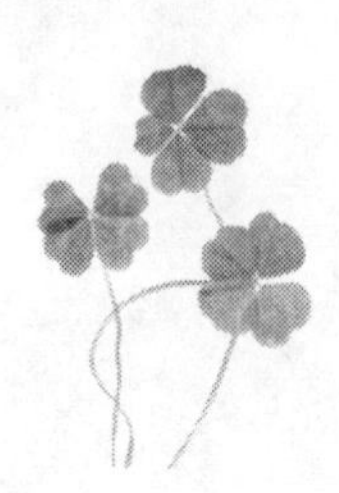

Ayurveda's unique contribution in the field of nutrition is monumental. In its forefront, lies the concept of the six tastes versus the four tastes that the modern human is most familiar with. Sweet, salty, sour, and pungent are the most common ones and relatively well known to us. But Ayurveda adds two tastes to the four above. It also includes bitter and astringent as tastes.

Picture your tongue and taste buds locations, and experiment with it and see for yourselves referring to the table and picture below.

Interestingly enough, each taste has a specific location which is associated with an organ that is most sensitive to the taste in question. The sensation in each area of the tastebuds also denotes the weakness or the strength of that particular organ respectively.

Picture 7.1: Diagram Tongue vs Organs vs Tastes

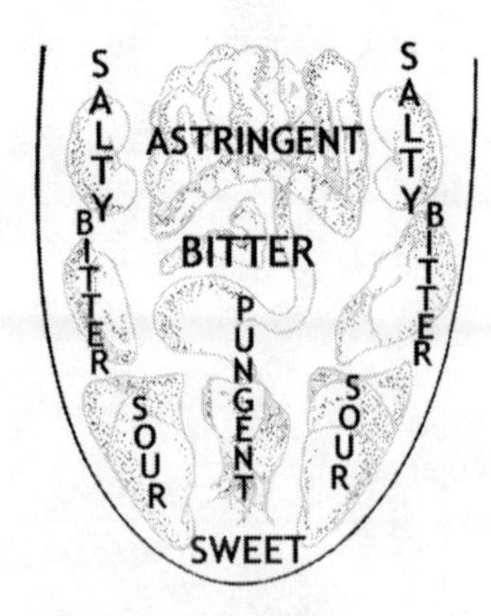

37 Rasas: a Sanskrit word means joy, pleasure, tastes applies to food and feelings alike

Table 7.1: Tastes vs Part of Tongue vs Organs

TASTES	PART OF TONGUE WHERE TASTE RESIDES	CORRESPONDING ORGANS
Sweet	Tip of tongue	Thyroid and apex of lungs
Sour	Anterior (front) part on sides	Lungs middle and upper lobes
Salty	Posterior (back) part on sides	Kidneys
Pungent	Front middle part	Stomach and small intestine
Bitter	Mid-part both side and middle	Liver on right, spleen and pancreas
Astringent	Posterior (back) middle part	Colon (large intestine)

The inability to sense certain tastes denotes an imbalance in the body. Having a clear grasp of the concept of tastes (the Rasas) and how to incorporate them into daily cooking will enable us to live ayurvedically in our daily lives. This is the prime objective behind this work: to help you, the reader, to become familiarized with the tastes in order to create balance. And this balance is not only in the physical body; it will enhance your mind so it can choose food options conducive to uplifting your spiritual tendencies.

According to Ayurveda, the concept of taste is not limited to what one may perceive in the first instant that something touches our tongue. Ayurvedic tastes enumerate and explore the first impact as the *Rasa,* meaning what it tastes like at the foremost. It may be enjoyable or repulsive, but regardless it triggers a response in us of sweet, sour, salty, pungent, bitter, or astringent. Then it moves to produce a reaction in our body that may be a heating or a cooling sensation. This is denoted as the *Virya*[38] of

38 Virya is the innate potency of the substance in question. It may be heating or cooling.

the substance in question. Thirdly, it has even further effect on our body and on our mind, which is the post-digestive effect denoted by its *Vipak*.[39] This shows us how it assimilates in our body-mind-spirit chemistry as either sweet, sour, or pungent and has a subtler impact on our well-being.

Some substances have a "miraculous healing effect" on our total well-being – one that is unexplainable in a way. This is denoted by the *Prabhava*[40] performing healing in the deeper levels of our tissues. This process of action/reaction/effect follows suit to everything that touches our tongue. Its applicability is the foundation of the Ayurvedic pharmacology of herb and spice usage in our daily diet and improves our culinary skills in the kitchen. With availing the know-how and applied knowledge of taste, one can create balance in a daily diet regime through the benefits of different substances. Foods provide us with gross nutrition, while herbs and spices provide the micro-nutrition at subtler levels.

Let us take an example of milk: The first taste of milk is its Rasa, which is sweet. The effect it has on our body is cooling, which is its Virya. Its post-digestive taste is sour, which is its Vipak. This will help you to see how mixing fruits and milk is contra-indicated, as most fruits end up in Vipak, which is sour or pungent. This results in increasing of sour tastes that will increase the acidic state in the stomach and intestine as a post-digestive effect. Increased acid state creates improper digestion which over- burdens the stomach which in turn end up creating toxins.

The same goes for yogurt which is sour in Rasa, even though it may feel cooling in Virya at a glance. But being sour in its Vipak increases the sour in the stomach, and this makes it contraband with any fruits as most fruits end up in sour post-digestive vipak. Going further, taking banana for instance: Its Rasa is sweet and astringent. Its Virya is cooling, owing to its Rasa. But its Vipak is sour, making it not the best to be combined

39 Vipaka is the effect that a substance has upon digestion in the small intestine; which can be sweet, sour, or pungent.

40 Prabhava is the special, hidden effect in a substance that is a healing response that is unexplainable and considered a "divine healing effect". Some foods and herbs, such as ghee and ginger root, have such an effect.

with dairy products as it renders our gastro-intestinal tract burdened with excessive sour post-digestive taste.

Therefore proper combining of foods with certain herbs and spices one can negate the negative effects and promote better absorption and assimilation. Ayurvedic cooking is therefore skilled with proper combination of foods to improve overall digestability of foods when combined together.

This is how the tastes enumerate in our gastro-intestinal tract and result in a healing or an aggravating effect. This knowledge will make us aware of what should or should not be combined to enhance the digesting ability of a substance. This is how Ayurveda helps us in applying its knowledge to benefit us in day-to-day food choices. Therefore proper food combining protects your digestive fires to function at its optimal best to benefit your overall total well-being.

Six Tastes

Each taste here represents its constitutional make up of its elemental nature present inherently in it. We explore each taste in a further detail.

The Sweet Taste

The word sweet brings many connotations to mind. In Sanskrit the original language of Ayurveda text, Sweet taste is '*madhur*' denotes; essence, joy, love, soothing, gratifying feelings owing to its elemental constituents of the earth and the water. Both its elements are the heaviest of the five elements. Therefore sweet taste tends to be heavy, cooling and oily in nature, and moves downward towards gravity in the body. When used in moderation it can promote grounding, satisfaction, vitality and strengthen the seven bodily tissues. It promotes the growth of plasma, blood, adipose fat, muscle tissue, bone, bone marrow and sexual fluids owing to its anabolic property.

The sweet taste quenches thirst and calms the burning sensation therefore enhances blood sugar. In moderation it is nutritive and healing, but in excess it can cause dullness and cause mal-functioning of the thyroid gland (refer the tongue / taste table). The sweet taste causes heaviness in the body and dulling of the mind which is cause of many other disorders. The sweet taste is the heaviest of the six tastes and makes blood viscous (thick) which can hinder a free flow causing congestion, diabetes, tumors, cysts etc

Foods which are strong in the sweet taste are molasses, honey, dates, figs, maple syrup, corn syrup, licorice root, marshmallow herb and root vegetable likes of potatoes, beets, turnips, sweet potatoes and pumpkin etc But in the mild hidden forms in the complex carbohydrate in the rice, ghee, wheat and most grains which are much slower in releasing their sugars.

It is now easy to see that sweet tastes therefore calms Vata dosha and Pitta dosha due to their light qualities, while it is aggravating to the heavy Kapha dosha. The sweet taste enhances the vital essence the 'Ojas[41]' which is the nectar from proper absorption and assimilation of foods we intake that strengthens the ability of procreation and boosts immunity.

The Sour Taste

Sour tastes are *Amla* and give a sharp, burning, heating, light, acidic, stimulating sensation owing to their elemental constituents of the earth and fire elements. It can be grounding for the vata dosha, but may aggravate the pitta dosha, while having a stimulating effect on kapha dosha. But it is stimulating to kapha only for a short-time usage. Any prolonged usage can aggravate the kapha dosha, owing to its earthy nature. Sour tastes stimulate digestive enzyme secretions and thereby stimulate the appetite.

Using sour taste moderately in the diet is essential for balance. It enhances the qualities of comprehension, appreciation, and discernment, but overuse can cause fermentation that leads to hyper-acidic conditions.

---

41 Ojas is the pure essence of kapha dosha and of the water element in particular.

That increases pitta in the body and mind and can flare up as various inflammatory conditions, such as skin rashes, psoriasis, hyper-acidity, excess thirst, heartburn, acid-reflux, anger, jealousy, and sour feelings like criticism, judgement, and rejection.

Sour taste denotes Vitamin C (ascorbic acid). It has the ability to burn fat in excess kapha conditions. As sour taste is most felt on the sides of the tongue, which is the location of the lungs, its overuse can have congestive effects on the lungs.

Its sharp, light, and burning qualities can promote alertness of the mind, but overuse can dry up the inner mucus lining. This can cause damage to the natural protective sheath of organ linings, thereby exposing the body to various inflammatory and congestive disorders.

Sour taste is often found abundant in lemons, oranges, grapefruits, vinegar, unripe mango, fermented foods, yogurt, sour cream, etc.

In mild forms in unripe fruits, and especially green lime (which is both sour and bitter), it makes a certainly superior choice of sour options for pitta and kapha dosha conditions.

The Salty Taste

Salty taste is *Lavana* and is heavy, hydrophilic, oily, and sharp, and has heating qualities owing to its elemental constitution of the water and fire elements. Its moderate usage calms the vata, but aggravates the pitta and the kapha dosha. Most commonly, salt exists in the form of sodium or potassium chlorides, which are the most common of salts in use.

The salty taste is most available in sea salt, rock salt, kelp (seaweed), and tamari. Ayurveda propagates use of rock mineral salts over common sea salt or table salts, owing to its mineral content making it a better health option. Although both sea salts and rock salt are salty in Rasa, heating in Virya, and sweet in Vipak, sea salts aggravate the kapha dosha. Hence, it is not the best option for hypertensive persons. This is due to *Prabhava effect* of the rock salts, which is a superior choice even for hypertensive conditions (but in moderation).

Owing to its elements of water and fire, it stimulates the digestive fire and makes food palatable by enhancing its tastes. The salty taste is anabolic in nature, promoting salvation and improving digestive enzyme secretions.

In moderation, it enhances absorption and assimilations processes. But in excess, it can lead to water retention and the depletion of body tissues, owing to its fiery and heavy watery qualities. We often loose body salts via sweat in hot summer seasons, and an increased intake of salty taste replenishes this vital element in the body.

In a balanced state, it maintains the body electrolyte balance. But in excess, it can cause water retention, skin afflictions, and edema due to increased pitta and kapha doshas. Due to a high intake of salt, blood become more viscous and this can lead to a thickening of the arteries that leads to narrowing of blood vessels and hence produces hypertension. That is the reason why people with high blood pressure are recommended to take low or even no salt in their diet. However, its scarcity can cause fatigued muscles.

In a balanced state, the salty taste enhances our spirit, makes us confident and enthusiastic, and boosts our healthy sense of self. While in the imbalanced state, it leads to dullness and a lack of creativity both in the body and mind. Our body produces twelve biochemical salts on its own. In depletion conditions, these can be supplied from the outside as readily available bio-chemical salts in health-food stores. It is a separate subject, but out of scope of this book.

Readers are welcome to explore this concept in *The Twelve Tissue Remedies of Schussler* by Boericke and Dewey.

The Pungent Taste

Pungent denotes *Katu* and constitutes the fire and the air elements. Owing to its constitutional elements, the pungent taste is heating, light, and dry in nature. Although as suggested by the elements it is pacifying to heavy kapha dosha, it can aggravate both the pitta and the vata doshas. In short-term usage, it can pacify all three doshas. However, in excess and over prolonged periods of usage, it will adversely affect both the vata and the pitta doshas. Therefore, discretion is important here: Those with pitta-dominant constitutions in hot summer months should be watchful of the pungent taste. Caution also needs to be maintained for keeping the vata in balance during the fall, when the vata dosha is high. While the kapha dosha can withstand long-term usage of the pungent taste, one should also keep the secondary dosha in the constitution in mind. If the secondary dosha is pitta, be cautious.

As the name suggests, pungent will assist in the kindling of Agni. Pungent taste is readily available via chillies (both red cayenne pepper and green hot chillies), black peppercorn, long black Pippali (piper longum), mustard greens and mustard seeds, horseradish, radishes, garlic, onion, and ginger to name a few.

Pungent taste activates both salivation and clears sinuses as seen by watery eyes when cutting an onion or eating green chillies. The sharpness of pungency helps in circulation, and hence is a natural blood thinner. It also helps in the breakdown of fat tissues, which helps to cleanse toxins from the body.

Moderation is the mantra to follow in Ayurveda – more is certainly not better. In excess, it can damage the body essence of the reproductive tissues in both males and females. Note that the male reproductive tissue (sperms) thrives in a cool environment. Therefore, excess heat through pungency in daily diets can render sperm less potent or even infertile. Excess consumption can cause strong thirst, burning, and/or anxiety. All inflammatory conditions are due to excess of pungent tastes. The protective layer of mucus membrane in the stomach can be damaged by excess use of pungent taste. Hence, it can result in various ulcerative inflammatory conditions. The pungent taste makes the blood and the body environment acidic. Therefore, it is contra-indicated for Cancer patients going through aggressive therapies like radiation and/or chemotherapy.

The pungent taste helps in the clearing of obstructions, bringing about clarity of the mind resulting in alertness, firmness, and determination. While being *rajasic* in nature can also make the mind become angry, aggressive, over-passionate, irritable, and envious, as well as incur jealous qualities. To cool off the anger and aggressive nature, use a little of the cooling sweet taste to bring about balance. That is the reason why a pitta prime constitution will/can crave for sweet tastes in the mid-afternoon – especially in the hot summer season. The sweet taste consumed at mid-day is easier for the body to process than when taken in the evening. As in the mid-day the digestive fire is more active than in the dark evening time when Sun is down.

I will make a special reference here to two unique herbs/spices: ginger root versus the Galangal root. Ginger is essentially pungent and sweet in Rasa, heating in Virya, and sweet in Vipak, thus having a further Prabhava of a sweet taste in post-digestion. This makes it the best friend for pitta dosha in spite of its pungency, *which makes it an exception to the rule.* Whereas, Galangal root, is essentially pungent in Rasa, heating in Virya, and *pungent in Vipak.* This makes it more pitta aggravating and an excess of it will have an adverse effect on the pitta constitution.

Another good example is hot cayenne pepper versus piper longum. Both spices are pungent in Rasa, heating in Virya, and have pungent Vipak. But piper longum changes its pungent Vipak to sweet Prabhava over the aging process. This quality of piper longum makes it safe for use for most pitta constitutions (even with hemorrhoids), while hot cayenne pepper is contra-indicated here for those with hemorrhoids.

The Bitter Taste

Bitter or *Tikta* constitutes the elements of air and ether. As both are light, cool, and dry in nature, they impart the same qualities to this taste. The Bitter taste increases the vata, but calms down both the pitta and the kapha doshas. Following the basic principle of Ayurveda – same increases same and opposite calms – the vata dosha is also made up of ether and air elements, making bitter taste extremely vata aggravating. Being the lightest of the six tastes, it has a drying effect on mucus, aiding the de-clogging of the body channels (the *Shrotas*[42]). On its own, it is not a very palatable taste, but it enhances the nutritional value of the foods we eat by making them bio- available and rendering them absorbable by thinning the saliva and melting the mucus.

Excess of bitter taste can cause emaciation and wasting of the body tissues due to its catabolic nature. But in conjunction with other tastes, it is a welcome asset. The bitter taste inhibits viral and bacterial growth, making it antibiotic by nature. All blood-cleansing herbs are bitter in nature. Yoga practices propagate the use of bitter taste. As its name indicates, it instils a quality of detachment in the aspirants. Slimming of the body makes one better able to practice yoga and lightness helps with fluidity during the yoga asanas. In excess, bitter taste can have a negative effect on the mind, promoting feelings of isolation and bitterness. But adding a certain portion of bitter tastes to the diet has some value as it can create suppleness in a being. But it only takes a little bit and the benefit can go a long way.

Foods that are bitter in taste are bitter-gourd (karela), fenugreek leaves, fenugreek seeds and sprouts, Arugula greens, and dandelion greens to name a few.

The Astringent Taste

Astringent or *Kashaya* constitutes the elements of air and earth. Owing to its elemental constituents, it tends to be cooling, dry, and heavy in nature. The astringent taste tends to reduce pitta and kapha dosha, but may increase vata dosha. The astringent taste causes a drying effect on the

---

42 Shrotas: are the body channels along which the vata –pitta--kapha doshas move from one part of the body to another. They are both physical channels and energetic channels and named 'Srotamsi denoting a river which starts as small then joins in with other channels to become a stream which flows becoming larger current. Many rivers meet the ocean same is true of the body channels many small channels come together to form larger Srotas, The Gastro-Intestinal tract is the largest of them all

tongue. A perfect example of this would be eating a raw banana, chiku, persimmon, or a pomegranate. One can add the astringent taste by eating green leafy vegetables like spinach, mustard greens, kale, and collard. Most vegetable and fruits are astringent in their un-ripe forms. All lentils and beans are a great source of the astringent taste.

The dryness of a astringent taste may even cause some to choke. The astringent taste absorbs excess moisture from stools and helps in proper formation of stools. But in excess, it can dry it up too much and may become an agent causing constipation and stagnation in the intestines and especially the colon. Therefore, in the case of loose stools, binding can be encouraged by taking an astringent herb like *kutaja*[43] or drinking buttermilk with 4:1 dilutions with water (four parts water to one part buttermilk), which is astringent.

Astringency by nature promotes healing in ulcers and inflammatory conditions. Mucus congestion can find relief with astringent herbs and spices like turmeric. Astringency promotes the drying up of open wounds and pus. Most facial masks contain astringent substances (like sandalwood and clay) to promote the drying of acne. In excess, it can cause aggregation and clotting owing to its drying qualities. Ayurvedic toothpastes are bitter and astringent compared to sweet conventional varieties that promote thinning of the saliva secretion. The bitterness and astringency aids in proper oral mastication of the food that helps a diabetic to have the proper breakdown of food in the mouth itself. The Ayurveda wisdom propagates that promoting proper chewing habits can help arrest the onset of diabetes at the mouth level. Therefore, teaching small children to chew their foods properly can drastically reduce the possibility of them developing

43 Kutaja is an astringent herb. Its Latin name is *Holarrhena antidysenterica*. Its bark, root, and seeds are used. It is bitter in Rasa, cool in Virya, and pungent in Vipak. It works well on digestive, excretory, and circulatory systems. It is astringent anthelmintic (kills worms, fungus, and bacteria) and amoebicidal (amoebic dysentery). Kutaja is specific to the colon in its action and helps restore its proper functions. It works very well for Candida conditions which is due to poor flora in the intestine, this herb helps to correct this. For bleeding hemorrhoids half teaspoon of Kutaja in half cup of pomegranate juice twice or thrice a day can do wonders to restrict bleeding

juvenile diabetes. Proper chewing can also instill mindful eating habits. At the mind level, an astringent taste has a grounding effect due to presence of the earth element. The grounded mind is able to meet daily challenges with a certain one pointed-ness. On the contrary, an excess of astringent taste can cause one to experience feelings like fear, anxiety, and nervousness owing to its air elements.

Elemental Constituents of Tastes

Ayurveda wisdom says: *You are not what you eat, but what you absorb."* Keeping this in the forefront, we enter the world of Rasas or taste. As mentioned in previous chapters, the importance of the elements in each entity applies here. Therefore, each taste owes its attributes and qualities to its elemental constituents. Each entity in this universe is bound by its elements, and each element in turn influences the nature of the entity in gross and subtle ways equally. The whole concept of nutrition and micronutrition is explained well through and through in Ayurveda.

Table 7.2 Tastes vs Elements vs Effect on Doshas

TASTE	ELEMENTAL CONSTITUENTS	EFFECT ON DOSHAS
Sweet (madhura)	Earth + Water	V ↓ P ↓ K ↑
Sour (amla)	Earth + Fire	V ↓ P ↑ K ↑
Salty (lavana)	Water + Fire	V ↓ P ↑ K↑
Pungent(katu)	Air + Fire	V ↑ P ↑ K ↓
Bitter (tikta)	Air + Ether	V ↑ P ↓ K ↓
Astringent (kashaya)	Air + Earth	V ↑ P ↓ K ↓

↑ Upward arrow denotes elevating or aggravating effect on the doshas

↓ Downward arrow denote pacifying or calming effect on the doshas

Clearly one can infer from the above table which three out of the six tastes calms a particular dosha and which three of the six tastes aggravate a particular dosha. The elemental make-up therefore delegates the effect a taste might have on our well-being at any given time.

Vata pacifying tastes are: sweet, salty, and sour

Vata aggravating tastes are: pungent, bitter, and astringent

Pitta pacifying tastes are: sweet, bitter, and astringent

Pitta aggravating tastes are: salty, and pungent

Kapha pacifying tastes are: pungent, bitter, and astringent

Kapha aggravating tastes are: sweet, salty, and sour

Each taste has its first experience at the tongue level and then in a deeper realm, where it is assimilated into the body. At that level, it creates a sense of balance, or when in excess, creates an imbalance that often surfaces as adverse cravings.

Ayurveda is the only holistic healing modality in which cravings are divided into healthy and non-healthy types. Healthy cravings are the body's own intelligence moving through to bring about a balance on its own. However, unhealthy cravings arise from unhealthy eating habits and a poor life-style in which the body has already produced enough toxins to cloud its normal cellular intelligence. This happens by avoiding certain tastes altogether as part of a daily diet. In essence, healthy cravings happen in the absence of toxins in the body, while unhealthy cravings are the direct result of the presence of toxins in the body.

When a body's inner-intelligence is clouded due to continuous deficient tastes, it in turn creates unhealthy cravings because of the nutritional deficit in the body. For example, choosing to eat hot spicy chillies in summer time for a pitta-dominant constitution; or eating cold, heavy ice-creams for a kapha-dominant individual in the dead of winter; or eating dry, raw, cold salads in the fall season for a vata-dominant constitution, is bound to create severe adverse side-effects over a period of time.

The body's own inner pharmacy is so accurate and precise, that it creates healthy cravings to create homeostasis (harmony) within the body. Have you ever had a cough and chills and craved black pepper or hot chilli or spicy ginger to help rid your body of the excess mucus? Have you ever wondered why a "hot cup of chicken noodle soup" hits the spot when you are sick in bed? The hot temperature soothes the chills, while the subtle pungent taste in the chicken has the capacity to give well-needed fat and nourishment and the noodle provides the much-needed energy for one to recuperate. Getting rest and having a light diet helps the body's own pharmacy to heal itself in a short time.

Often we ignore the warning signs our body is sending us for much-needed rest to allow our body do its own healing. Instead, we opt to reach for the quick fix of a cold and flu remedy, and keep eating and continuing to go to work as if nothing is wrong. Doing this causes the body to be sick longer with more side effects that take longer to heal.

Did you ever wonder why when mucus clogs the tongue you fail to really taste the essence of the food and have no desire to eat? You've probably noticed that as you recover from being sick, you also recover your sense of taste and your appetite revives. Believe it or not, this is your body's own innate intelligence at work here. Fasting is natural tendency of your body's own internal healing response. The appetite is the first thing that makes a comeback when balance is restored within the body. Therefore, Ayurveda states that if you have healthy appetite, eliminate regularly, and sleep well, you are likely healthy.

The secret behind the culinary art of Ayurvedic cuisine is the incorporation of all six tastes in the meal. This will bring about a healthy essence to all bodily tissues, a sound mind, and a joyous integrated spirit. Thus, it is natural for an Ayurvedic practitioner to be an ardent cook with a sound knowledge of food items and the healing qualities of various spices and herbs. These provide the micro-nutrition essential for enhancing the absorption and assimilation processes in the body-mind-spirit.

Any food item can be rendered more palatable and absorbable with incorporation of the simple Ayurvedic principles of *gunas* (qualities innate in foods, herbs, spices, mind, and spirit). Applying this knowledge and basic principles can and will result in helping you balance and replenish the body, mind, and spirit so you can sustain a balanced state and enjoy the simple joy of good health. It is lot simpler than it is made out to be.

Table 7.3 Doshas vs Daily Cycle vs Life Span Cycle vs Seasonal Cycles

DOSHAS	24-HOUR CYCLE VS DOSHA	LIFE SPAN VS DOSHAS	SEASSONS VS DOSHAS
Vata	2 to 6 a.m. and p.m.	50+ years	Fall and pre-winter
Pitta	10 to 2 a.m. and p.m.	25 to 50 years	Late-spring-summer
Kapha	6 to 10 a.m. and p.m.	Birth to pre-teen	Winter and early spring

To conclude, we live under the influences of cycles: The day and night cycle is governed by the three bio-energies, the aging process is governed by the doshas, and the changing seasons also have doshas predomination. Using this wisdom, one can live easily in harmony and respect each stage, each time of day, and each seasonal cycle as it aligns with natural laws.

When we ignore these cycles and laws, we pay the price for the omissions of our own innate intelligence. With this clear look at tastes, we are now equipped to move forward and go deeper within our bodies to see how the process of digestion is influenced by these six tastes through the six stages in the digestive processes.

Chapter Eight

The Six Stages Of The Digestion Process Congruent To The Six Tastes

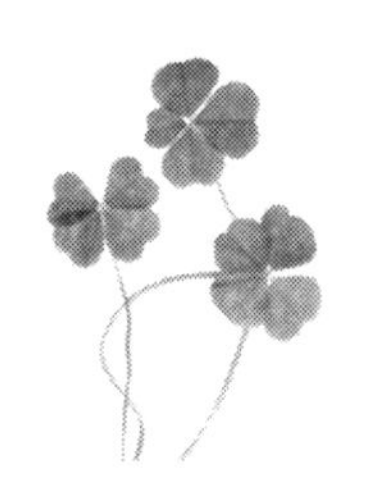

"A healing diet gladdens the heart, nourishes the body, and revives memory."

—Sushruta

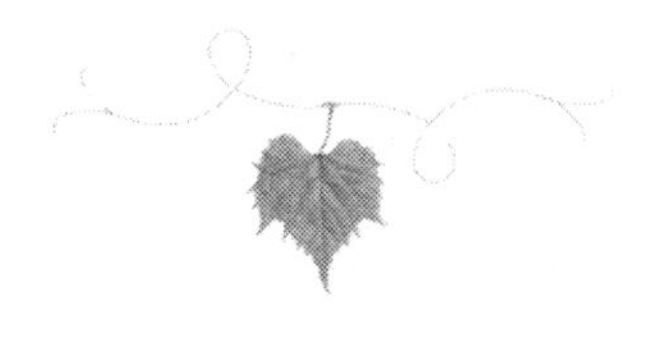

Six Stages of Digestion through the Gastro-intestinal Tract

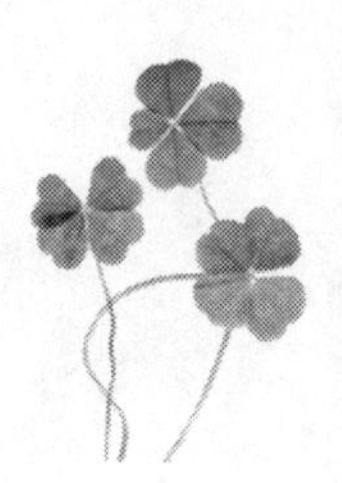

The importance of foods to nourish our body tissues, the mind, and the consciousness is the foundation of Ayurvedic nutrition. Simple foods are nourishing and healing to our whole *Being*. They maintain health at each level of our physical bodies, mental bodies, and ethereal bodies. This foundation makes up the stage for realizing deeper realities of the total human experience.

Ayurveda propagates the Truth that has survived over millenniums from times immortal. It's time-tested authenticity needs no further proof. This truth is simply waiting to be explored by the curious, inquisitive minds of the modern day. *It is clear that a single cell carries within itself the whole recipe for its re-creation.* It is also true to say that *each seed holds the tree within.* Likewise, we hold the secrets of the whole cosmos within us. Finding the secret will undoubtedly set us free. This freedom is the doorway to Salvation.

The three dynamic forces of nature, creation, sustenance and dissolution are operating constantly all around us from eternity to eternity. It is reality that nature is a continuum standing witness to the wisdom of the ages of which we are an important part. We are not here accidentally. We have a definite purpose and reason why we are here as did the first seed born out of the womb of nature (the Cosmic Mother) and nurtured by the warmth of the Sun (the Cosmic Father) water and wind. It carried the cosmic memory to create and recreate itself. Today, it is continuing to do the same right in front of our eyes. Can you see it? Our body is living proof of this testimonial – that our body regenerates its ownself on a regular basis. We are not the same as the day we were born, but essentially what makes us into US? It is worthwhile to ask this question.

Our body cells are continuously dying, regenerating, and changing. Look at a picture of you from your early years and compare it to one of you today. Even though it is not the same you, you "know" it is indeed you. What is in you that "knows" without any shadow of a doubt? Exploration into Ayurveda can take you to the answers within for sure.

The five great elements form the foundation of the tripod of the three bio-energies of the tridoshas. The tridoshas in conjunction with the ten pairs of opposing qualities *(the gunas)* form the six tastes. The six tastes form the foundation of the process of digestion through its intrinsic qualities of Rasa, Virya, and Vipaka that are applicable to all foods and medicines alike. Finally Vipaka of *specific miraculous effect* gives some foods and substances their *Prabhava* that gives the concept of Ayurvedic nutrition its uniqueness.

We experience the first taste (Rasa) in our mouths when our tongue touches the substance. This initial taste is felt as one of the six tastes – either sweet, sour, salty, pungent, bitter, or astringent. Once it reaches the stomach and small intestine it clearly generates its effect showing its quality and potent energy, the Virya. The Virya works through the effect of digestive enzymes on the substance. The effect generally is of heating or cooling. Everything in nature has its own innate qualities that cannot be separated from the substance. For example, fire has the quality of heat and light innate within it, and this can never change. The same is true with the coolness in the snow. Therefore the Virya of a substance – be it of heating or cooling – has a direct effect on the state of the digestive fire (Agni).

Heating Virya stimulates pitta but pacifies both vata and kapha doshas. Heating kindles digestive fire/enzymes, raises body temperature, and therefore, enhances circulation. But in excess, it can burn vital tissues and its essence, the Ojas. Due to its hot and sharp qualities, it promotes catabolic activity (depleting qualities) causing ulcers, inflammatory diseases, and bleeding disorders.

Cooling Virya pacifies pitta dosha, but may aggravate vata and kapha doshas. Cooling nature is anabolic (promotes growth) and may douse the digestive fire (low Agni) and decrease the body temperature. With excessive and long-term use, it will cause a low metabolic rate and poor digestion and assimilation, creating metabolic toxins in the body and the mind.

Sweet taste is cooling in Virya, but there are exceptions to this rule: Honey and molasses, even though sweet, can be heating. Lemons generally are sour, making it heating, but the bitter/sour of green lime renders it cooling. These exceptions are due to the Prabhava initiating a healing response to various areas of the body.

As general rule of thumb, sweet taste is the most cooling when compared to the cooling of bitter and astringent tastes. Sour and salty both are heating, but sour proves to be more heating as compared to salty owing to its elemental (fire and water) content.

The Virya upon moving through the intestines in the gastro-intestinal tract creates its post-digestive effect called the Vipaka. The Vipaka takes place in the colon where it directly has effect on the stool, urine, and sweat. Liver enzymes play a role in creating the Vipaka of a substance by its action on them. Ayurveda enumerates three types of Vipaka: Generally, sweet and salty tastes (Rasa) generate sweet Vipaka, sour (Rasa) taste generates sour Vipaka, and bitter, pungent, and astringent (Rasa) tastes have a pungent Vipaka. Exceptions to the rules are owing to the Prabhava effect.

The sweet Vipaka is anabolic and increases the kapha dosha by adding bulk, which can also promote dullness. While the sour Vipaka triggers an increase in digestive fire, hence affecting the metabolic activity by increasing the pitta. Lastly, pungent Vipaka has a strong catabolic (depletion) affect, owing to its drying qualities that can increase the vata.

The Prabhava of a substance is the *awareness in action of innate cellular intelligence* that cannot be explained. For example, "clarified butter" known as "ghee" taken with warm milk in the quantity of two teaspoons in one cup of milk acts as a laxative, while one teaspoon dose in one cup warm milk acts as constipating. The Prabhava is credited here – the innate intelligence inherent in the substance that creates certain unexplainable healing responses in the body-mind chemistry.

The foods we intake undergo the digestion process with the aid of the digestive fire (Agni) present in the digestive enzymes. Once digested by the enzymatic action, it is absorbed and assimilated to provide well-needed energy for each aspect of our growth. Each stage in the digestion process has a distinct taste associated with it. Hence, digestion has all the tastes in its food contents – sweet, sour, salty, pungent, bitter, and astringent. As food passes through each stage via enzymatic actions, it attains its predominant taste. Thus, digested food becomes the base for all deeper tissue assimilation. The key organs in the process of digestion are: the saliva in the mouth, insulin from the pancreas, liver enzymes, bile secretions from the gall bladder, etc. Digestion, therefore, helps in breaking down the complex foods into simpler absorbable forms that can be easily assimilated by our bodies.

Each part of the digestion process is as good as its Agni. If digestive fires are weak, the process will not be efficiently executed. Agni is present in each enzyme, the doshas, sub-doshas[44] (each doshas has 5 sub-doshas), and the deep body tissues. Each level has its own processing Agni. Malfunction on any level of Agni can and will lead to indigestion. This can result in the accumulation of the metabolic toxins (Aam) in the body.

One must remember here that each of the three doshas has their individual functions. For example, the vata's function is to provide mobility so foods can move through the body within the cells, out of cells, cell to cell, and out of the body. The pitta's function is to assist by secretions of the metabolic enzymes that are essential in and for all metabolic functions. Lastly, the kapha's functions are to maintain the integrity of the cell walls and provide lubrication for the easy flow of nutrients during the digestive process.

---

44 Vata, pitta, kapha doshas are each further subdivided into five sub-doshas, signifying the 5 great elements, according to their location in the body. The five vata sub-doshas are: Prana, Udana, Samana, Apana, and Vyana. The five pitta sub-doshas are: Pachaka Pitta, Ranjaka Pitta, Sadhaka Pitta, Alochaka Pitta, and Bhrajaka Pitta. The five kapha sub-doshas are Kledaka Kapha, Avalambaka Kapha, Bodhaka Kapha, Tarpaka Kapha, and Shleshaka Kapha,

Table 8.1 Digestion Stage vs Taste vs Element vs Organ vs Tissues vs Dosha

STAGE	TASTE	ELEMENT	ORGAN	TISSUES	TIME	DOSHA
First	Sweet	Water and earth	Mouth and upper stomach	Plasma	First hour	Kapha
Second	Sour	Fire and earth	(Fundus) Lower stomach	Blood	Second hour	Kapha
Third	Salty	Water and fire	Duodenum	First muscle and second adipose fat	Third to fourth hour	Pitta
Fourth	Pungent	Air and fire	Small Intestine	bone	Fourth and part of the fifth hour	Pitta
Fifth	Bitter	Air and ether	Ileum	Bone marrow	Sixth hour	Vata
Sixth	Astringent	Air and earth	Colon	Semen and ovum	Sixth to seventh hour	Vata

The six stages that food passes through in the digestion process usually take six to eight hours. One taste relates to each stage of this digestion process. Each taste strengthens the next stage by its processing. The foods usually falls under basic four types: soups, solids that you need to chew, drinks, and licking kinds like pickles or ice cream.

The aroma and sight of the food stimulates the appropriate brain centres and the digestion begins even before food makes its way into the mouth.

The first stage in the digestion process happens in the mouth itself when we chew our foods. The digestion of the carbohydrates begins in the mouth through the action of ptyalin (enzyme) in the saliva of the mouth. Saliva is one of the sub-doshas of the kapha (the bodhaka kapha; the mucus) that helps in the easy swallowing of the food through the food pipe and enhances the taste perception of the foods.

Saliva maintains the electrolyte balance and temperature in the oral cavity. Healthy thin saliva denotes happy mind; a dry mouth is a sign of ill health as we often see in fear, anxiety, and stress. Thick mucus excess is due to the malfunction of the pancreas and can indicate an early onset of diabetes. Young children often drool a lot as they are in prime kapha age and are generally happy and joyful. Saliva also maintains healthy flora of the mouth by killing bad bacteria. The Ayurvedic life-style encourages brushing teeth and scraping the tongue first thing in the morning to eliminate the dead bacteria from the mouth. The scraping positively effects and massages the various internal organs to work optimally. Food passing through the esophagus enters the stomach.

In the stomach, food undergoes further churning. The churning of the food with the help of the stomach enzymes makes food further liquefied. The activity of the stomach mucus, stomach enzymes (pitta), and stomach air (Samana-vayu) initiates further breakdown of the bigger food molecules to further simplify. The first hour of the digestion process is the "sweet stage" in which the sweet taste is processed, even though the food has all the other tastes in it. The fundus part of the stomach secretes enzymes through its mucosal lining that completely change foods to a fine liquid form. The simple sugars are digested here and immediately released into the body to provide instant satisfaction and energy. The stomach is one of the most elastic muscles in our body. It can expand well to accommodate large portions of foods. This stage provides the ground for nourishing the first body tissue, the rasa-dhatu. Its prime function is to bring a sense of contentment and nourishment.

The second stage in the digestion process is the "sour stage". The sour taste is made up of earth and fire elements. The food here continues to break down to even a smaller and finer texture. The heaviness of the initial hour becomes lighter in this stage due to fire element in the sour stage. The stomach environment is sour due to the secretion of hydrochloric acid through the smaller curvature of the stomach. The mucus present in the stomach (the Kledaka Kapha) acts as a protective layer. This kapha-mucosal lining acts as protection to stop the acid here from eating up the stomach itself. In eating excessive hot foods, this lining gets damaged and can cause heartburn, gastritis, gastric ulcers, and various other inflammatory conditions. The sour stage is a pitta-increasing stage by its nature. Therefore, excessively consuming sour taste in a diet will cause an increased risk and exposure to bouts of hives, rashes, itchiness, and eczema.

In this sour stage, the hormone gastrin stimulates secretion of the enzyme pepsin. Pepsin starts working on the protein part in the foods, whereas the enzyme rennin secreted in this stage acts on milk-protein by coagulating it. This is seen more so in infants than in adults. The second stage nourishes the second body tissue which is the blood tissue (the Rakta-Dhatu).

The third stage of digestion process is the "salty" stage, when food enters the duodenum (the first part of the small intestines). The food here is emulsified by the secretions from the gall bladder and the pancreas. The bile secreted from the gall bladder and the pancreatic enzymes secreted from the pancreas are both alkaline in nature. Here the alkaline juices meet with the food coming from the stomach, which is acidic. This chemical reaction between the acid and the alkali results in formation of salt and water. The salty stage acts further on digesting both the proteins and fats in the foods. The enzymes amylase, trypsin, and lipase are part of the pancreatic juices. This stage of the digestion process nourishes the third body tissue, muscle tissue, and the fourth body tissue, adipose fat – the Mamsa-Dhatu and the Meda-Dhatu respectively.

The fourth stage in the digestion process is the "pungent stage". It takes place in the latter part of the small intestine, the jejunum. The air and fire elements predominate this stage. The fire element changes the colour of the food in this stage to yellow then to brown. In this stage, the pitta increases in the body. An excess of pungent taste in the diet can lead to skin rashes, hemorrhoids, and bleeding disorders. Air is important for absorption of nutrients to nourish the next body tissue, the bone tissue (the Asthi Dhatu). The strength of the peristaltic movements in this latter part of the small intestine determines the quality of absorption. Any malfunction at this stage can cause various indigestion disorders that generate metabolic toxins. The metabolic toxins coat the intestines and hinder the absorption of nutrients into the body. One may eat all kinds of nutritious organic foods, but if your body has toxins in the small intestine it will be hindered in the absorption process.

The fifth stage in the digestion process is the "bitter stage", which takes place in the ileum, the latter part of the small intestine. The presence of bile salts in this part of the intestine makes the food bitter. The dominance of air and ether elements helps in maximizing the absorption of nutrients through the villi in the inner wall lining of the small intestine. The air element also helps in the peristaltic movement (vata aspect) to continuously push the food to the next part of the process. In this stage, one might feel light, creating a false sense of hunger although the digestion process is still not complete as yet. The food still has not gone through the astringent stage. The end product of this stage nourishes the bone and bone marrow tissues (the Asthi Ddhatu and the Majja Dhatu). The movement of the sub-doshas of vata dosha opens the ileocecal valve pushing the food into the cecum. The cecum is the first part of the large intestine. In the cecum, the food changes to astringent.

The sixth and the final stage is the "astringent stage" that takes place in the cecum, the ascending colon, and part of the transverse colon. The elements of air and earth are dominant in this stage of the digestion process. Air helps in the movement and earth forms the bulk of the end product of digestion. The astringent quality here promotes the peristaltic activity. When the food passes through the second part of the transverse colon, maximum amounts of the fluids are passed through to the kidneys to be eliminated as urine. The food forms the bulk of fecal matter as it passes down the descending colon to the sigmoid colon. The downward moving Vayu (the Apana Vayu) helps in the movement of the fecal matter out of the body and initiates the elimination process. The astringent taste nourishes the reproductive tissues, hence completing the six stages of the digestion process. The colon is the prime site of vata and keeping it functioning optimally will help balance the vata dosha throughout the body.

The timing of the digestion process may vary from person to person. It is influenced by the constitution of an individual. It is said that in approximately six to 8 hours, the six tastes nourish the formation of the six unstable, immature forms of the body tissues. Further, each immature tissue takes approximately five days to mature to its stable form. The full maturation of the seven body tissues takes a total of 35 days. Therefore, in approximately 35 days, the final body tissues and reproductive tissues are formed. You may be wondering here and ask if what we eat today will form the healthy reproductive tissue in 35 days? The answer is: Yes, it does take 35 days to produce healthy reproductive tissues. This is the very reason why it is suggested to follow any food, medicine, or dietary change for a period of 35 to 40 days for its full effectiveness.

Ayurvedic nutrition is therefore complete and whole in its applicability. It needs nothing added or removed to render it complete. The choices we make with the nature of the foods we intake and its due processing in return nourishes not just our physical, but also mental and ethereal bodies as well.

Once we as humans discover ourselves fully, all other secrets of the cosmos shall unfold on their own to us. Birth, life, and death are part and parcel of the total human experience. But only a few of us get to the real depth of realizing and fully awakening to the true purpose of life. The wisdom contained in Ayurveda provides us with the sound foundation on which we can comfortably rest our journey to explore within. The foods we consume lie at the forefront of this journey. Its importance is clearly narrated in the ancient texts of Ayurveda just waiting to be unfolded by us.

Only seeds that are left alone and are pristine pure can grow healthy plants. The healthy plants have the power to positively affect our body, mind, emotions, and feelings. Therefore we must take special care to choose the best of the best that nature has to offer. If undermining this power of nature, the human race has to face its wrath.

Chapter Nine
The Wonder Foods That Can Rescue You: Nature's best Healers

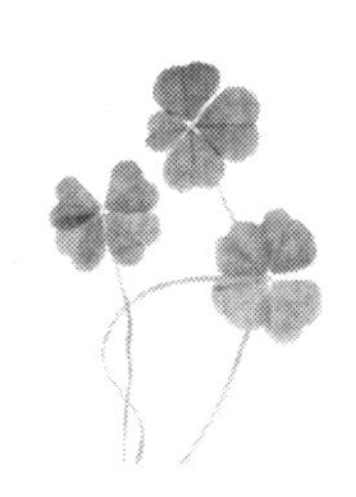

"The entire world seeks food. It is the life source of all beings. Clarity, longevity, intelligence, happiness, contentment, strength, and knowledge are all rooted in food."

—Charaka

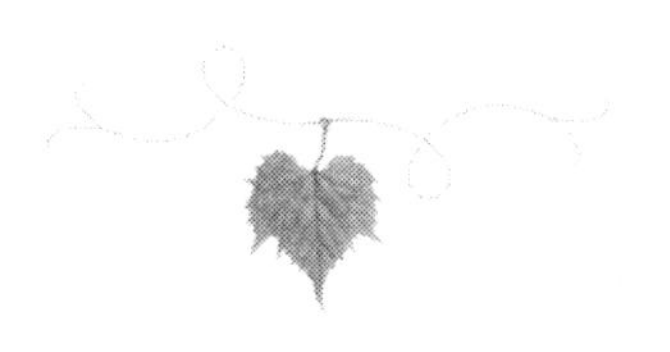

The Foods We Consume Become the Consciousness We Are

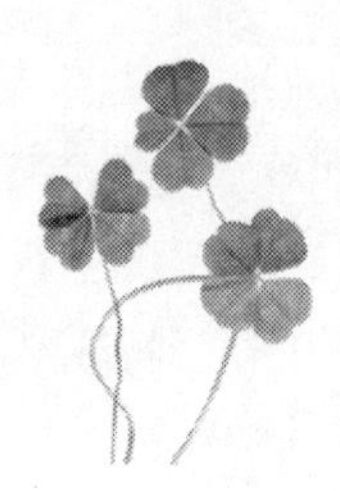

Food is everyone's basic need. We consume food to nourish our body, grow, and prosper. Food is more than nutrition. Digestion and nutrition are subtle processes that transform foods into consciousness. Foods are the gross forms of subtle energies. The foods we choose have an influence on how we will nourish our bodies and nurture our minds to enliven our spirits.

The question to ask is: How do we know what we are eating is the best of foods? Simple, pure natural foods – ones that remain untouched by human hands and are unaltered by any further modifications – can be considered as good foods to consume. Those foods that are grown on fertile lands with natural resources will produce healthy produce. The quality of the land, processing, harvesting, and retailing all play a very important part in the quality of foods we receive in our supermarkets today.

The Ayurveda texts designate certain foods as healing foods. Wholesome seeds carry the memory of their origin and are nourished by the five great elements. When we consume such foods, they in turn nourish our five elements in a wholesome way. All foods – may it be a plant, shrub, tree, herb, fruit or seed – possess the life-giving nectar, its *Rasas*. When we consume such foods we benefit from their healing properties.

In Ayurveda, foods are divided into three types: High-quality foods like milk, ghee, rice, wheat and fruits that are sweet, cooling, and calming to the mind are the *Sattvic* foods in nature. The heating and stimulating foods like pepper, ginger, radish, hot and spicy foods, are the *Rajasic* foods in nature. And heavy, debilitating, non-nourishing, stale and old leftover foods, garlic, alcohol, and ice creams are considered the *Tamasic* foods in nature. We can develop our cognitive memories by understanding that certain foods affect our bodies and minds in a positive and/or negative way.

In this chapter, we will talk a little bit about certain wonder foods from the text, *Charaka- Samhita* that were identified as the first foods of the earth. These foods have been in use by humans for millenniums and continue to nourish us by their healing qualities to date.

These are foods such as rice, barley, grains, mung beans, amalaki (Indian gooseberry) fruits, rainwater, rock salt, honey, milk, and ghee. Animals and birds, such as grey partridge and common quail that habited dry forests, all served as supplements to this original diet as narrated in the Ayurveda doctrines.

The grains were the most sustainable primary foods. Each civilization has witnessed their value thus far. Rice is considered the "king of grains" as it has provided well-needed complex carbohydrates since the beginning of times. Wheat and barley were considered the more cooling of the grains as compared to millet, quinoa, rye, with buckwheat as the most heating. One must choose grains that are the most beneficial for our constitution. Among lentils and beans, green mung beans are the "queen of legumes" and are the most beneficial of all. Legumes provide our diet with necessary protein. Most beans are astringent in nature providing an important taste for the body. The larger the beans, the longer it will take to cook, hence they are also harder to digest. Therefore, smaller beans that are fairly easy and quick to cook with little processing are the most nutritious and easy to digest.

Be aware and tuned to the fact that something good may not be good for YOU. Always be aware how certain foods do not agree with you and certain are like nectar for you. One person's nectar could be other person's poison. Therefore eat according to and conducive to your own constitution. But foods that are prepared with all six tastes will stand a better chance at being a balancing food for all constitution types.

Let us now look into some wonder foods that deserve a mention here as we explore our best food options. May it guide you, the reader, to add them in your diet to reap their benefits for your optimal health. I have chosen the following five great wonders: amalaki fruit, ginger root, honey, ghee, and aloe vera. This is meant to be a prelude to the next book in this series on Ayurvedic nutrition.

Amalaki Fruit: The Natural Complete Wonder Fruit

Amalaki Fruit
Common name: Indian gooseberry
Latin name: *Emblica officinalis* Family: *Euphorbiaceae*

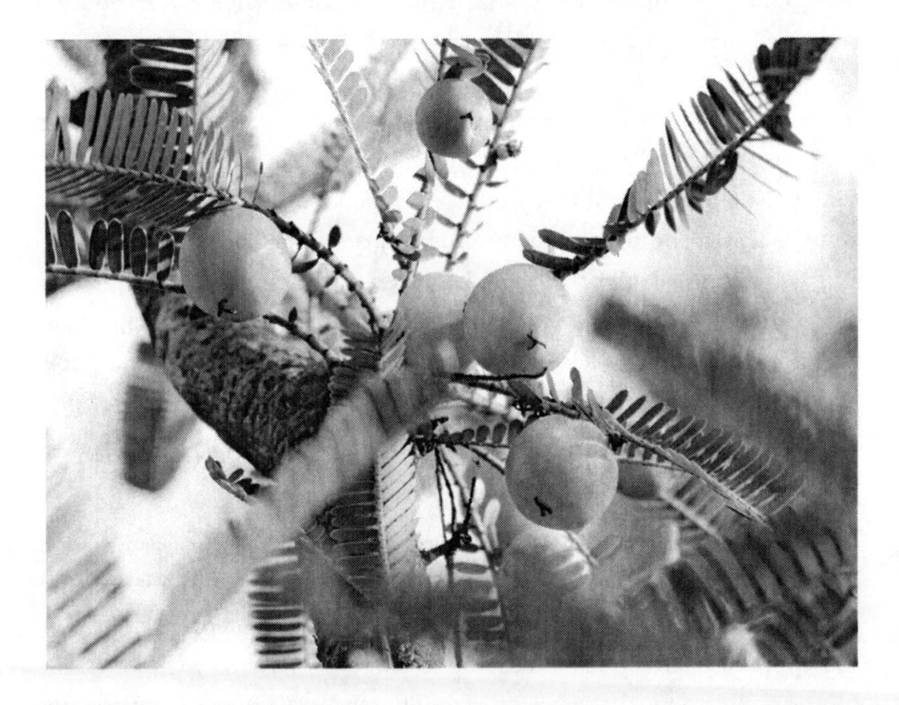

Picture 9.1: Amalaki Tree with Fruits

Amalaki (the Indian gooseberry) is one of the most ancient foods on this planet. The Amalaki is a tree, which grows in Asia and bears small lemon-sized fruits for several months in a year. The Amalaki fruit contains five of the six tastes that Ayurveda propagates. It is missing only the salty taste, earning itself the glory of being as complete and perfect food a human can consume provided by Mother Nature.

It is sweet, sour, bitter, astringent, and pungent in Rasa, cooling in Virya, and sweet in Vipak. It works on all body tissues and increases vital energy, the Ojas. It is not advisable to eat it raw, but cooking renders it most palatable. Its juice can be added to other fresh vegetable and fruit juice preparations.

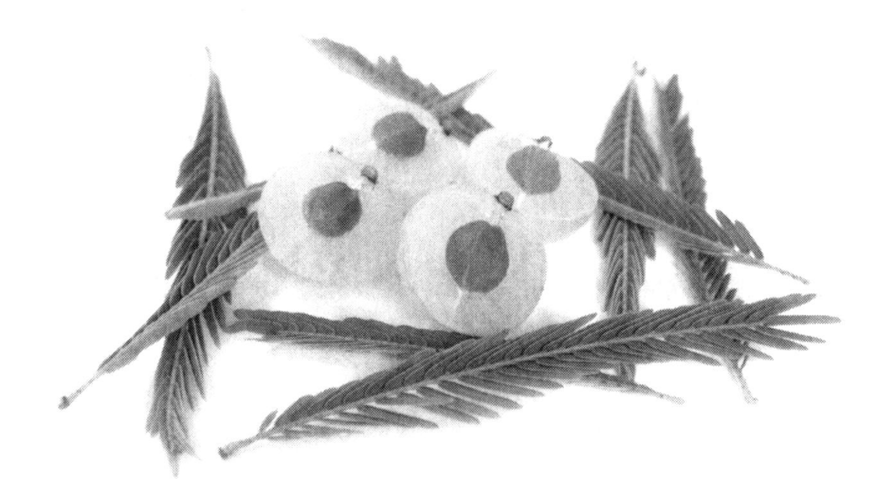

Picture 9.2: Amla Fruit

It is most beneficial in bleeding disorders, hemorrhoids, anemia, diabetes, constipation, weakness in the liver and spleen, hair loss, and rejuvenation. It is also the best immune booster.

The Amalaki fruit improves the appetite; it is cleansing to the intestines and regulates blood sugar. It is one of the three main ingredients in a popular Ayurvedic preparation known as the *Triphala*.'[45]

The amla fruit as it is commonly known is naturally divided into five segments holding the significance of the five elements. The Amalaki fruit is extensively used in Ayurvedic medicines. This fruit is most beneficial as a great source of Vitamin C, making it the most powerful anti-oxidant

45 "Tri" means "three" and "phala" means "fruits". Thus, triphala is a combination of three fruits: Amalaki (Emblic Myrobalan), Bibhitaki (Beleric Myrobalan) and Haritaki (Chebulic Myrobalan). Triphala is the best laxative and bowel tonic and balanced rejuvenator in Ayurvedic medicine.

money can buy. The Vitamin C contained in it is heat resistant, making it a stable immune booster and a rejuvenator. It is said that one fruit has the equivalent Vitamin C of 20 oranges or 10 limes (approximately 3000 mg/fruit). It retains its efficacy even after due processing. Due to its high potency, small amounts can be sufficient.

It is beneficial for all three doshas, but especially for pitta constitution. It is usually available fresh in most East Indian grocers. It is one of the key ingredients in the most popular Ayurvedic preparations called the *Chyavan Prash*, a rejuvenating herbal jelly preparation. It is sattvic in quality. It is one of the best mind tonics.

Ginger Root: The Cure-all Medicine

Ginger Root
Common Sanskrit name: Adarak
Latin name: *Zingiber officinale* Family: *Zingiberaceae*

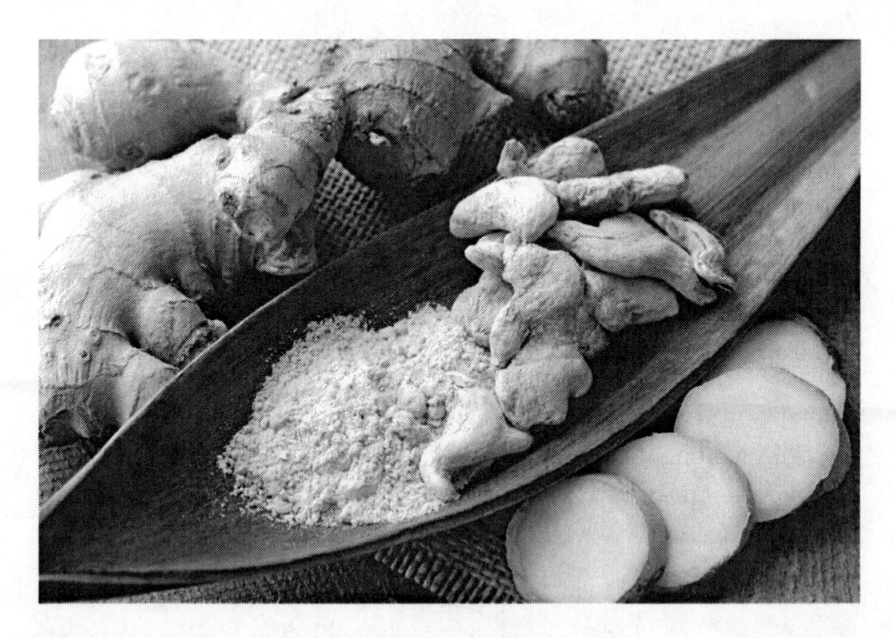

Picture 9.3: Ginger Roots & Powdered Ginger

A native of Southeast Asia, the ginger plant is a perennial creeper with a thick hardy rhizome producing an erect annual stem. At the end of the stem grows greenish purple flowers. This root carries the earth's fire, making it pungent in Rasa, heating in Virya, with a sweet Vipak as the post-digestive taste.

In its dry form it is called S*unthi*, but in fresh form it is called *adraka*.

In Ayurveda texts, it is mentioned as a *Vishvabhesaja,*[46]meaning a universal medicine fit for any ailment. Although pungent and heating, it is sattvic in nature and induces peace. The rhizome root is the most beneficial part of the plant. The ginger root is an excellent cardiac tonic and digestive stimulant. When used with lime juice and honey, it provides excellent relief for anorexia by stimulating a healthy appetite while scraping the body of excess mucus. When used in lime juice with rock salt, it promotes digestion. It is very common in an East Indian home to have a bottle with ginger/lime juice/rock salt preparation sitting permanently on the dining table at meal times.

It is beneficial and widely used in treating colds, coughs, indigestion, nausea, hemorrhoids, and headaches, as well as in purgation therapy (induced elimination). Although it is best for vata and kapha disorders, it is safe for pitta to avail of its benefits owing to its sweet Vipak and special Prabhava (innate beneficial effect), thus making it one of the safest tri-doshic remedies of all times.

It is easily available at grocery stores worldwide as a result of globalization. It can be eaten in its raw form, juiced, or used in cooking. Its usage is open to your own creativity. So go ahead and explore.

---

46 Vishvabhesaja comes from "vishva", meaning "universe" and "bhesaja", meaning a cure-all. Thus it is a universal cure-all for all ailments.

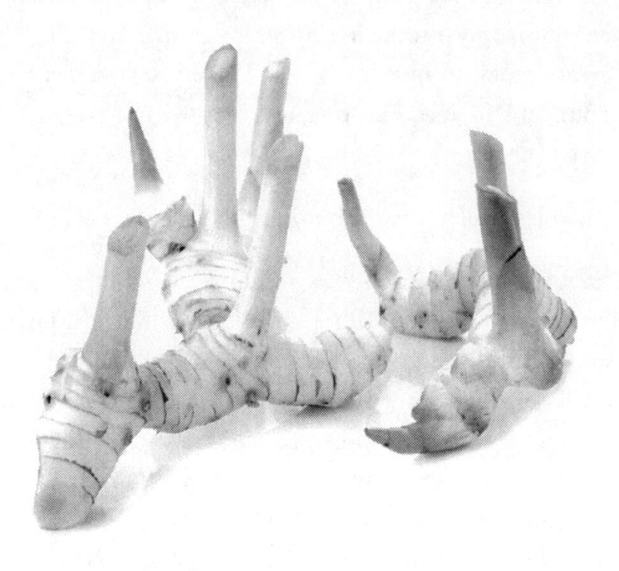

Picture 9.4: Galangal Root Rhizome

Latin name: *Alpinia officinarum* Family: *Zingaberaceae*

Its sister look-alike herb is called Galangal root. Looks can be deceiving, so be informed before using. It is a rhizome used in Thailand by the natives as a culinary herb. The Galangal has tighter and lighter skin and is pinkish in color. It is more like a pepper than ginger. Both grow underground and can be interchanged in recipes, but energetically both are different. Galangal is pungent in Rasa, heating in Virya, and pungent in Vipak, while ginger is pungent and sweet in Rasa, heating in Virya, but sweet in Vipak.

Making use of ginger root is far more superior to galangal in its utilities and healing properties. The Galangal is popular in Thailand, Indonesia, and China. Ginger is most popular in India. Globalization and its popularity have made this herb easily available worldwide.

Honey: Mother Nature's Best Gift

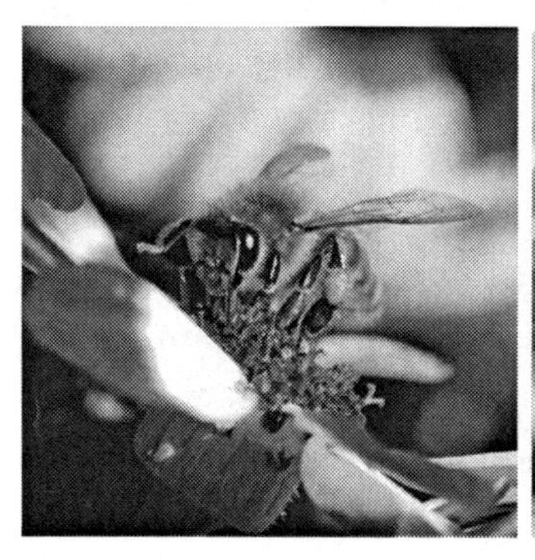
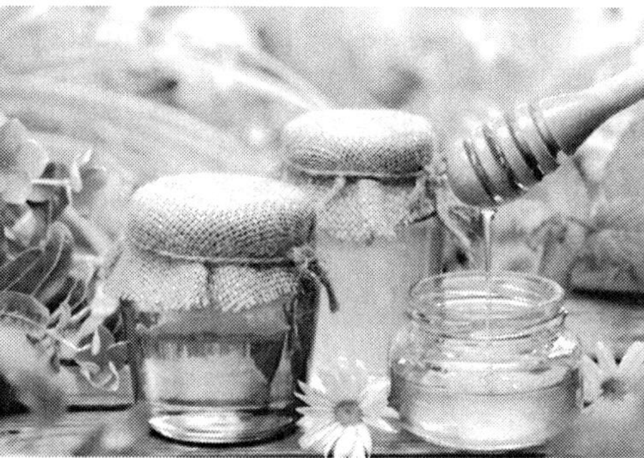

Picture 9.5 Flower & Honey Bees
Picture 9.6 Pure Unpasteurized Honey

Honeybees are the world's best organized and dedicated creatures from whom we can learn much about creativity and selfless labour. Beehives symbolize harmony, sisterhood and brotherhood. Honey is Mother Nature's simple gift to humankind. It is a pre-digested food made by nature that our body can easily assimilate without requiring much processing by the body. Honey is a complex substance made up of mostly fructose and glucose with traces of minerals, some vitamins, no fat or protein, and small amounts of sucrose. It has not only the sugars from the nectar of flowers, but also some "additives" from the digestive systems of our friendly bees. These additives act as the preservatives in honey, maintaining its freshness for long periods of time. It is sweet, pungent, and astringent in Rasa, heating in Virya, and sweet in Vipak. It can be used as an expectorant, emollient, nutritive tonic, and laxative. It is calming for vata and kapha, owing to its heating quality, but in excess can aggravate pitta.

It is considered nature's nectar as it gives life to the lifeless, rejuvenates the elderly, and provides strength to the weak. It is beneficial from infancy through to old age. A clean natural source of warmth and energy, it is laced with certain vitamins in trace forms, such as Vitamin B1, B2, Vitamin C, Vitamin B6, pantothenic and nicotinic acids. Besides carbohydrate and vitamins, it is rich in some hormones. In eastern cultures, it is the first food put on a newborn infant's palate. However, on the contrary in conventional medicine it is not advised to give newborn infants under the age of one year to be put on honey. I leave to your own discretion to choose.

Honey made from different flowers in different regions differs in taste and colour. The regional quality of the air and water influences its colour, aroma, and taste. Light colour flowers usually yield light colour honey with sweet fragrances. Mustard flowers render a yellow colour of honey. The thickness and thinness of honey depends on the season in which the nectar is collected. Bio-chemically, honey contains acetic acid and malic acid along with traces of citric, famic, lactic, phosphoric, tartaric, butyric, capric, caprylric and amino acid in traces, to name a few. Honey is well laced with enzymes like diastase, invertase, catalase, inulase, maritalm and dalsitol. Nectar collected from the stigma of a flower also adds some protein and nitrogen into the honey. The fragrance of honey is due to colloidian from the nectar of flowers. The colloids are similar to protein molecules present in honey 1-9%. Upon closer look, it is evident how honey molecules are similar to our own DNA molecule. But going into detail on each constituent in honey is beyond the scope of this book. However, I have tried to put forward a picture that will encourage you to research into it in a deeper way.

Our friends, the honeybees, collect nectar from approximately 62,000 flowers to make up one kilogram of honey. For each half kilogram of honey, honeybees go out about 3,700,000 times.

Each beehive can have up to 75, 000 bees working tirelessly. Once the hive is full, bees will close the hive with a wax-like secretion, thus closing it neatly, as if protecting their own hard work by sealing it.

Each flower has its own healing qualities that are then transferred into the honey. Honey kills germs owing to its hygroscopic nature. The high sugar content and astringent nature draws the life giving water out of any germ, killing it in the process and promoting healing.

Honey is widely used all over India, Germany, and Europe for the variety of its healing properties for treating burns, typhoid fever, acne, and even cancer. It is still used as a "healing spread" on hard-to-heal open wounds to date. It is useful in promoting weight gain in slim people, as well as to melt away excess fat in the obese. It is a natural tonic.

In India newborns are given a drop of honey on the tongue before putting them on the breasts, it increases the amount a child drinks from the mother and results in a healthier baby. Toddlers are also put on Indian unleavened bread and honey as their first foods before starting on vegetables and other foods. The sweet taste is everyone favourite and induces anabolic activity, hence encouraging weight gain in the initial years of an infant's life.

Fresh honey is heavier and more difficult to digest. But the older it gets, the lighter and more healing it becomes. Due to its complex nature of carbohydrates, honey is delicate and easily damaged with heat. Therefore, honey should be consumed raw in the unpasteurized form. Any heat processing renders honey toxic. Therefore cooking with honey is not recommended, although it can be added to foods after they are cooked. It can be put in warm water, but not on direct heat. Equal quantities of honey and ghee is considered toxic according to Ayurvedic texts. But mixing one part of honey to three parts of ghee is nourishing and healing. It is used as a vehicle when mixed with herbs for delivering the healing qualities of the herbs to the deeper tissues.

Honey when used in diet as a sweetener has advantages over other sugars. It is absorbed relatively slowly due to its high fructose content. The kapha constitution should avoid sweeteners in teas, with the exception of honey. All sweeteners are good for pitta except honey. All sweeteners are good for vata as it helps balance out the vata-increasing properties of the other foods and herbs.

Are you wondering how does one know if the honey they are using is pure? Try this simple test at home: Take a clear glass and fill it up with water at room temperature, then add a drop of honey into the water. If the drop settles at the bottom without dispersing midway, it is pure honey. But if it disperses, it is not pure.

It is not uncommon to see that after a certain period some varieties of honey get crystallized. Often some remains a thick liquid on the top portion, while lower portions get crystallized. Some varieties of honey that do not crystallize have less grape sugars and more fruit sugars. Honey that does not crystallize is beneficial for diabetics. Generally crystallization is common in good varieties of honey, as this shows its purity. It is a myth that such honey is harmful and has sugar contamination. Some honey farmers think that such honey will not sell well, so they tend to heat it prior to bottling it so it will not crystallize on standing. However, this process kills certain beneficial constituents in honey, so be aware. Honey that looks like a thick spread is perfectly fine to consume. In summer months, it tends to become liquid and soft, while in the winter, it can thicken up more.

Honey is food, medicine, and sweet all in one. Consuming it can never harm you, and only benefit you. However, other sugar products available on the market are certainly harmful. Many foods are laced with such hidden sugars that you do not even suspect. Therefore, becoming well informed can help you to make a conscious choice to avail of honey's benefits fully.

Recently I had an opportunity to visit and meet with a lovely couple who run a local honey farm in Ontario, Canada. I invite you to explore and visit them for premium quality, unpasteurized honey and to support our local farmers in the process. **Visit them at RAE's Honey House. Owners: Glenn and Diana Rae, Box 169, Holland Centre, Ontario, Canada, NOH 1R0 (1-519-794-0939).**

Ghee: Divine Elixir

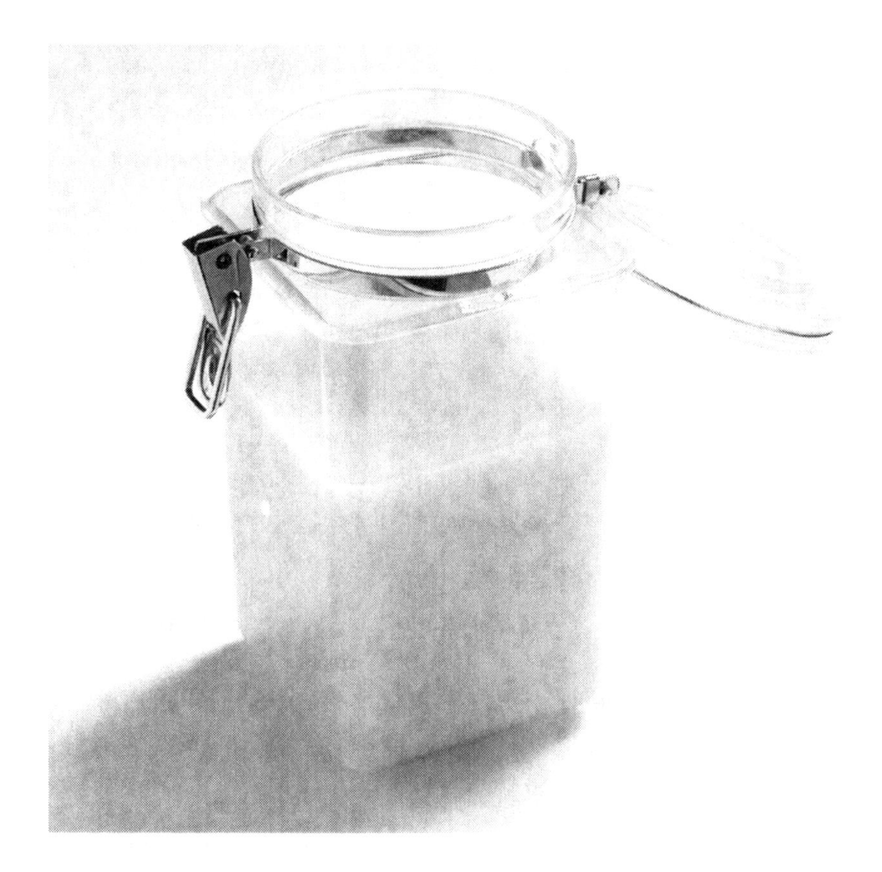

Picture 9.7 Ghee in the Jar

The cow in East Indian traditions is considered a life-giving holy animal that nourishes us like a mother nourishes its child. A lactating mother produces milk from the food she consumes in the same way that cows assimilate grass and convert it into milk for us. Humans are the only species on this planet that drink milk from another species other than its own after infancy. As per nature, each animal only feeds its own offspring. The cow is worshipped as a "Mother" in India by the natives to date.

From cow's milk comes butter, yogurt, buttermilk, and ghee. Milk is a sattvic food as long as it remains untouched and unaltered. The quality of the milk a cow generates depends greatly on what kind of food the cow is grazing on. The higher the quality of grazing foods is, the higher the quality of the milk. Such milk will yield good quality butter. The best quality butter will make the best quality ghee. How well the butter is then processed and stored greatly influences the vitality of the resulting ghee, just as a breastfeeding mother has to take utmost care in her daily diet to make up the best quality of breast milk for her young infant.

The Ayurvedic texts have praised ghee for centuries. The *Sushruta* (first Ayurvedic Surgeon) regarded ghee as an intelligence-promoting principle when used appropriately in the body, while the Sage *Charaka* has praised its glory and said, "Ghee made from the best quality of cow's milk has the ability to promote both memory and the vital bodily essence, the Ojas."

Ghee is considered the most vital of the dairy medicines, associated with the element of love in the body. On its own, or added to herbs, it is widely used in Ayurvedic formulations. Organic milk yields the best quality butter, yogurt, and ghee.

Ghee is a sweet, cool, light, and oily food. The Ayurvedic texts mentions ghee as a *Agnivardhak*[47] – a substance that promotes digestive fire, and *Yogavahini*[48] – a substance that takes on the properties of the foods and herbs that it is mixed with, thereby acting as a vehicle to transport the healing essence of the herbs to the deeper tissues.

Today's milk unfortunately is not of the best quality. Most farmers are using poisons, chemicals, antibiotics, hormones, and arsenic stimulants to increase milk production. This has rendered the supply poor in nutrient value. The state in which the animals are kept and handled is something to be looked into as well. The fear and torture these innocent animals are put through has greatly affected the milk supply of today. When we

---

47 Agnivardhak comes from "agni", meaning "fire", and "Vardhak", meaning "to promote or ignite". Thus, Agnivardhak is a substances that promote the digestive fire.

48 Yogavahini comes from "yoga", meaning "joining" and "vahini", meaning a "vehicle". Thus yogavahini is a quality whereby the healing quality of foods, spices, and herbs can travel through the medium of ghee and promote the betterment of health.

consume such milk laced with all sorts of additives and stimulants, they find their way into our human bodies as well.

Thankfully, some recent efforts have made by many independent farmers globally to commit to producing good quality milk and milk products that are free from hormones and pesticides. Many family-owned farms are feeding their herds of goats and cows with feed that is free of such harmful chemicals. We owe our ardent gratitude to them all. We as citizens of this world must encourage such efforts more and more.

Organic ghee, free of chemicals, hormones, antibiotics, and GMO's is among the best. Ghee is made by boiling butter on a slow fire to evaporate the milk solids. (Refer to the recipe in Appendix VI of this book.) The water in the butter has live enzymes that encourage bacterial growth. Boiling it evaporates the water, leaving behind the pure fat form that is pure ghee. It is also called "clarified butter" by many French culinary experts. Note that properly made ghee does not require refrigeration. The ghee is resistant to scorching as it is free from water, while butter burns on cooking. It is a lot easier to cook with ghee than with butter. The best culinary preparations and many French dishes use "clarified butter".

Ghee blends well with other foods and helps to make them more bioavailable into the deeper tissues. Ghee promotes the formation of the essence of food known as Ojas, therefore making ghee at home is a healing practice. Ghee is tri-doshic, but is most beneficial to vata and pitta doshas.

In modern context, ghee made from cow's milk butter is made up of cholesterol and saturated fat and is a semi-solid at room temperature. Whether it increases bad cholesterol levels and triglycerides or accumulates the chemicals found in butter on the market is currently not known. But hundreds of years ago, when no other fat was available, ghee was the prime source of fat used in all cooking in India. The longevity and health of individuals at that time were far better than today. Diabetes and heart diseases were hardly ever heard of in past centuries. Whereas today, diabetes and heart disease are reaching epidemic proportions in India and abroad.

I leave it to readers to use the statistics available to make a viable decision regarding their use of ghee, the divine elixir, in their diets.

The Butyric acid found in saturated fats is known to inhibit the growth of tumors. The role of healthy cholesterol in the maintenance of healthy brain functions, nerves, and liver functions is also no secret. It is a fact that our brain is thirty percent fat and all the nerve cells are coated and protected by a fat-layer called the myelin sheath. This shows how a good fat can be essential for optimal health. The function of kapha in the body is essential for cellular integrity. The Ayurveda texts clearly indicate its importance in maintaining healthy levels of tissue and organ functional integrity.

In ghee, the key ingredient is CLA-conjugated linoleic acid, which in recent studies has been shown to slow down the progress of certain cancer and heart diseases and may also be responsible in reducing body fat while increasing lean mass. Usage of any substance with proper understanding of its benefits and with discretion will provide maximum benefits to the aspirant.

Organic ghee promotes spiritual energy. Spirituality is the subtlest form of nutrition and is only available through certain foods. Ghee is one of them, earning its glory as "the divine elixir". Ghee benefits all three doshas, but kapha constitutions need to observe caution as they are fairly well lubricated already. Ghee is easier to digest and aids absorption of other nutrients in a way regular butter cannot. Ghee builds marrow, semen, and ojas, and improves intelligence, memory, vision, voice, and digestion. It nourishes major organs, such as the lungs, liver, kidney, and brain.

Ghee promotes longevity. It is very calming and nurturing for the elderly, as well as for young children. It is lactose-free, which is beneficial to those who are lactose intolerance. The milk solids are evaporated and discarded during the making of ghee. Ghee is used both internally and externally in various Ayurvedic *snehana*[49] therapies and mixed with different Ayurvedic

---

49 Snehana are lubricating, loving therapies where oiling of the body promotes calming of vata and pitta doshas. When oil/ghee is mixed with herbs, it increases its benefits many fold.

herbs. Internal application promotes cleansing of bodily tissues and the elimination of excess doshas. The medicated ghees are used in various conditions, such as peptic ulcers, skin afflictions, blood disorders, insomnia, epilepsy, paraplegia, tumors. etc. The various medicated ghee preparations are called the *ghritas* and are used both internally as well as externally in therapies. I have listed a few of the popular ones in the table below for readers' benefits.

Table 9.1 Ghritas (Medicated Herbal Ghee) vs Benefits vs Herb Used

GHRITAS	BENEFITS IN	HERBS USED
Tikta and Mahatikita ghee (bitter + alterative herbs) Barberry ghee	Skin and blood disorders	Bitter tasting herbs, katuka, neem, gentian, manjishta barberry, alterative herbs
Brahmi ghee Bhringaraj ghee Saffron ghee Basil ghee	Mental afflictions	Brahmi Gotu-Kola, Bhringaraj Saffron Basil
Gugullu-tikta ghee	Muscular pains, cholesterol management	Guggulu-resin with bitter herbs
Ashwagandha ghee Shatavari ghee Saffron ghee	Vitality tonic, fetal tonic	Ashwagandha Shatavari Saffron

Aloe Vera: A Total Healing Panacea

Common Binomial name: AloeVera
Aloe spp,; Family *Liliaceae*
Sanskrit name: Kumari, meaning a young girl or virgin.
Aloe is so called because it imparts the energy of a youth
and brings about the renewal of the female nature.

It is a succulent plant and part of lily family (Liliaceae), the same family that garlic and onions belong to.

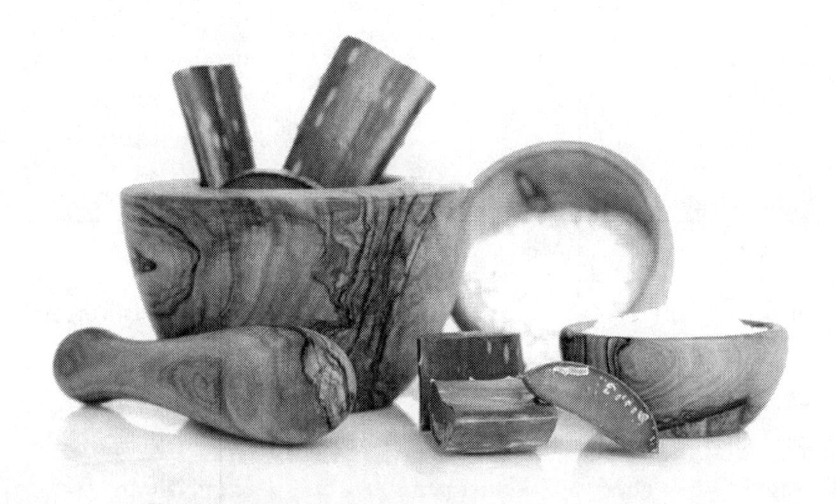

Picture 9.8 Aloe Vera Plant and Usage

The Aloe plant is known as the "Queen of the Dessert". This plant grows in the dry, sunny terrains of South-eastern and Northern Africa, India, Spain, Indonesia, and the Caribbean. Most recently its popularity has spread to Australia and the United States. It has been used medicinally for centuries by the East Indians, Chinese, Greeks, and Egyptians.

It is a cactus with succulent thick leaves filled with a gel-like sap that is a natural tonic for liver, spleen, blood, and the female reproductive system.

It is bitter, astringent, pungent, and sweet in Rasa, cooling in Virya, and sweet in Vipak. It works on all tissues.

Aloe is a wonder food that has variety of benefits to its credit. It is an excellent blood cleanser. It is a mild laxative, which regulates the intestinal peristaltic movements. It promotes digestion and relieves abdominal distension by promoting downward movement of the wind. It helps all three doshas. It is especially useful in pitta disorders like fevers, skin afflictions, acne, burns, peptic ulcers, hemorrhoids, menopausal symptoms, insect bites, sunburns, and edema, to name just a few. Aloe vera primarily works on the thyroid gland, pituitary gland, and ovaries. Therefore, aloe regulates the fat and sugar metabolism and tones the Agni.

It is an overall rejuvenator and skin toner and is calming and softening to body tissues. It is used both in douching therapies and herbal enemas. It removes parasites from the colon and improves its flora.

It is more palatable when taken mixed in water or apple/cranberry juices. The raw form is stronger in action than the commercial variety, which is much more diluted. As a tonic it can be combined with the herb *Shatavari*[50] as a bitter tonic with the herb *Gentian*,[51] to regulate menstruation along with the herb *Manjishta* [52]. Externally its gel can be applied topically to sunburn, burns, sores, herpes sores, etc. However, refrain from using it during pregnancy and in uterine bleeding.

---

50 Shatavari comes from the Sanskrit word which means "who possesses a hundred husbands." Latin name: ***Asparagus racemosus***. Family: ***Liliaceae***. It is a tonic and rejuvenating to female reproductive organs and circulatory, respiratory and digestive systems. It is especially good for pitta dosha.

51 Gentian is a classic of bitter herb which helps destroy Aam, the metabolic toxins, in fever and inflammatory conditions like genital herpes and cancer. It works on blood, plasma, muscle, and fat tissues, as well as on both digestive and circulatory systems.

52 Manjishta is a root which is the best alterative and blood purifying herb in Ayurvedic medicine. It works well on the female reproductive system and circulatory system. Its ability to dissolve obstruction extends to the liver and kidney too.

Conclusion

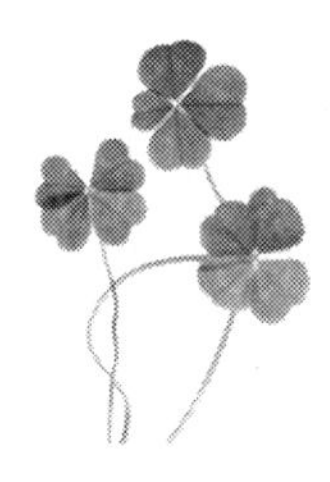

"That person who always eats wholesome food, enjoys a regular lifestyle, remains unattached to the objects of the senses, gives and forgives, loves truth, and serves others, is without disease."

—Vagbhata Sutrasthana

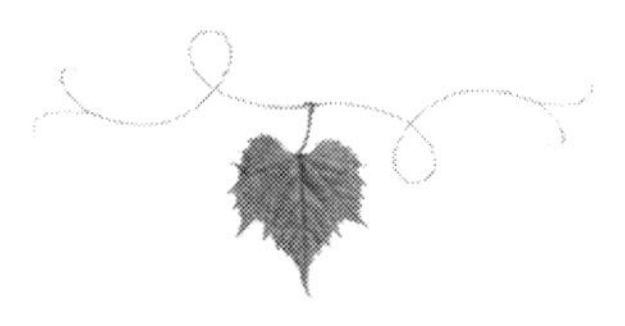

Ayurveda's age-old wisdom is pure and pristine owing to its adaptability to changing times and needs. Its viability is beyond questioning as it is time-tested wisdom. May the reader find the content here enough to create more thirst and hunger in them to explore it further in their lives. This is the first step towards a never-ending journey. By reading it, you have taken that first step. Come let us walk together to further explore. I remain a perpetual student to this eternal medicine that heals all unselfishly and whole-heartedly.

Deepening The Understanding: Review Questions

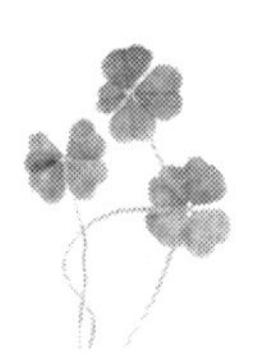

Chapter One Review Questions
The Ancient Wisdom: A Gift To Humankind

Test yourself by exploring the following questions:

1. How must one approach one's endeavours in life? Is there an end to one's own journey within oneself?
2. What is Ayurveda?
3. Where did it originate from and when?
4. How is today's human different from his predecessor?
5. How did our ancestors live?
6. Is it a true that "Old is Gold"? Support your answer.
7. How was the knowledge of the art of living imparted to humankind? By whom and to whom?
8. Are we better off today than our ancestors? Explain

9. How has Ayurveda maintained its relevance through the challenge of changing times?

10. Is Ayurveda relevant today to modern human? Can it rescue us today?

11. Would you choose what Ayurveda has to offer you today? How can it help you personally?

12. What is "our birth right"?

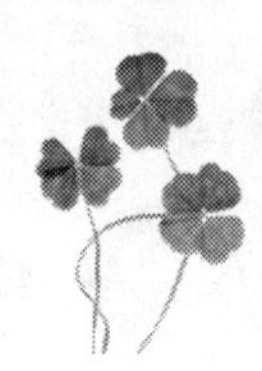

Chapter Two Review Questions
The Birth Of Ayurveda: The Theory Of Creation

Test yourself by exploring the following questions:

1. How did the world we know today come about?
2. What are the two most important aspects involved in the creation process? Explain their nature and roles.
3. Are we limited to our physical bodies?
4. What entities in this universe are the building blocks that connect everything to everyone?
5. Who is the proponent of "The Theory of Creation"?
6. What are the key components in "The Sankhya Model of Creation"?
7. What is the main principle of the enumeration process?
8. What are the "Great Elements"?
9. What are the Sanskrit names of the great elements?
10. What are the Tanmatras? What is their relationship to the "Five Great Elements"?
11. Which element is subtlest and which is grossest and why?
12. Which element is responsible for transformations in the external and internal worlds?
13. In which element's presence can the rest of the elements exist and why?

14. Which element is responsible for sense of smell?
15. Which element is responsible for sense of touch?
16. What element makes taste possible?
17. To what element can we credit our sense of hearing?
18. Did you know your elemental reality before you read this? How has it benefited you knowing it?
19. How are you different than this book you are reading and how you are same? Explain.

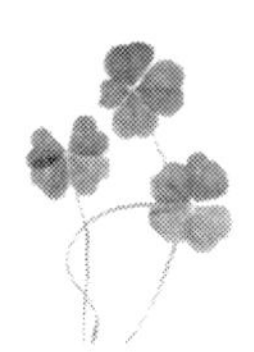

Chapter Three Review Questions
The Great Elements: The "Panch-Maha Bhutas"

Test yourself by exploring the following questions:

1. What is the essence of existence?
2. What is the nature of Space (the ether element)?
3. Which element is home to all others?
4. What form of energy is associated with the element of ether?
5. Directional ether takes the form of which element?
6. What is the subtle essence of the air element called?
7. What are the attributes of the air element and how do they benefit us in our body functions?
8. What is control of breath called in terms of Yoga? How is it beneficial to us?
9. "In absence of this element no movement is possible." What is this element? Explain why you agree or disagree with this statement.
10. Which element carries all transformational changes in the body and nature?
11. The discriminative quality is attributed to which element?
12. What form of energy is associated with fire?
13. How and why is the element of water significant for us?

14. Can we live without water? Why? Support your answer.
15. Which element is the heaviest of them all?
16. Which element is the lightest of them all?
17. What physical symptoms occur during an imbalance in the earth element in our bodies? Why?
18. What mental qualities might one display if he/she had an imbalance of fire elements? ★Bonus marks: Give one example of a case when it is high and one when it is low?
19. Do all the elements remain the same all through the year? Support your answer with an example of which element influences:
    a. Summer season
    b. Fall season
    c. Spring season
    d. Winter season
    e. Rainy season
20. Are your diet and lifestyle influenced by changing seasons? Explain why?
21. Malfunctions of which element is responsible for Alzheimer?
22. What are Doshas? How do they come about? How many are they? What are their names?
23. ★Ulcers are more prone to which Dosha? Bonus Marks★
24. ★Tumors are common in which Dosha? Bonus Marks★
25. ★Anxiety and fear will occur more so in which Dosha? Bonus Marks★
26. Which direction does the water element move in and why?
27. Which direction do the ether and air elements move in and why?
28. What element is rough, cold, and dry?
29. What is most important for your survival? Why?
    a. Food
    b. Water
    c. Air
30. What is the most popular course of treatment in Ayurveda for cleansing and nutritive purposes?
31. Which of the treatments is not available in North America but still practised in India?

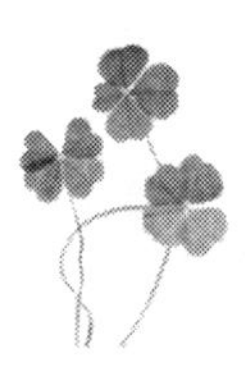

Chapter Four Review Questions
The Qualities In Nature And Matter:
The "Gunas Attributes"

Test yourself by exploring the following questions:

1. What are the qualities inherent in nature?
2. How is the 24-hour day divided into these qualities?
3. What quality prevails in infant stage?
4. What quality is prominent in old age?
5. What are the attributes of matter in nature?
6. How can one use the knowledge of attributes to balance oneself?
7. What is the nature of the summer season?
8. What is the nature of early spring? If you are sick with heavy mucus in this season, what quality will give you relief and why?
9. What qualities does warm soup have?
10. Green chillies belong to which attribute?
11. An anxious mind has what attribute?
12. A stubborn nature denotes what quality?
13. A blissful state reflects which attribute?
14. What time of day is most Sattvic?
15. What is Rajasic time?
16. What is good about Tamasic quality?
17. Most dense foods are also _________?
18. A 16-year-old girl is having trouble motivating herself to get out of bed and go about her day. What do you think is happening to her, and what would you suggest to help her to take charge and live optimally and enjoy life?
    a. Which quality is making her the way she is at present?
    b. Is this a permanent state for her?

c. Adding or taking out which qualities will improve and bring changes in her situation?

19. Which attributes carry tamasic, rajasic, and sattvic qualities? Give example from foods and state of mind qualities for each one.
20. What do you call your present state of health? Is it different from how you were when you were born? If yes, what caused the change? And what can you do to bring about a balance if needed? Explain briefly.
21. Explain the division of attributes in a twenty-four hour cycle?
22. If you are 60 years plus, what part of your life span are you in? Explain.
23. What stage of your life is the Sattvic by nature?
24. What times of the day are Rajasic and at which stage in your life is it reflected the most?
25. How do the knowledge and wisdom contained in Ayurveda help your life? What would you like to change in your daily regime that you haven't before now?
26. What is the Ayurvedic Mantra regarding attributes?
27. How does the nature of food and its attributes effect your health?
28. Can Ayurvedic wisdom be applied by anyone anywhere? Explain how.
29. . If you are a 35-year-old woman or a man, what diseases will you most likely be afflicted with at this stage of your life? Why?
30. What are the ten pairs of opposites according to Ayurveda? Give an example for each pair?

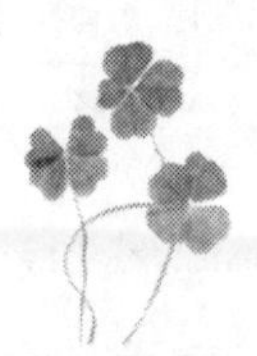

Chapter Five Review Questions The Tridoshas: The Tripod Of Ayurveda – "You Are Unique" Says Ayurveda

Test yourself by exploring the following questions:

1. What results in interaction between the great elements? Explain.
2. What are Tridoshas? What are their innate qualities?
3. How do Tridoshas form the foundation of who you are?
4. What is constitution?
5. Can two people with the same constitution be considered the same? Explain.
6. What is Vikruti?
7. What are the body characteristics of a Vata individual?
8. What are the mental characteristics of a Pitta individual?
9. Slow and steady fits which type of individual?
10. Fast and furious fits which type of individual?
11. Changing and uncertainty is innate to which type of individual? Why?
12. If your prime dosha is Vata which job will best suit you? Why?
    a. Flight attendant
    b. Order picker at a warehouse
    c. Assembly-line worker
    d. Retail store attendant
13. If I am a Kapha prime, which food option is best for me for breakfast? Why?
    a. Milk and yogurt items
    b. Fresh fruit, like papaya and pear
    c. Dry cereals with goat milk
    d. Eggs
    e. Black coffee
14. If I am a Pitta prime and Vata secondary (PV) individual, which season is most pacifying and why? Which is the most aggravating and why?
    a. Fall season
    b. Summer season
    c. Winter season
15. If I have a medium frame, love to eat sweets in the afternoon, and like to get up and go in the mornings, which type am I? Why? But when I eat hot chillies, I get a _______? (pimple, rash, or hemorrhoids)
16. When I was born, I had curly hair and I bit my nails all the time. Which type am I? Explain your choice.
17. What is always constant in me, never changes, and defines my es-

sence?

18. What constantly changes in me through the day, seasons, and my ages?
19. What is the main goal of an Ayurvedic consultation? Explain?
20. Who can benefit from such a consultation and why?

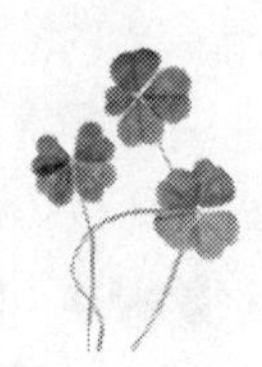

Chapter Six Review Questions
The Digestive Fires: The Concept Of "Agni"

Test yourself by exploring the following questions:

1. What is the significance of "Agni"?
2. What role does it play in our health and ageing process?
3. How can one protect his/her own "agni"?
4. What is the source of "agni" in external nature and its internal counterpart inside our body?
5. What are the signs that show poor functioning of "Agni"? Give examples.
6. How does one know one's state of good "Agni"?
7. What is death in terms of Ayurveda?
8. What are Dhatus and Malas?
9. How can one enhance functioning of "Agni"?
10. Name one herb that can rekindle poor "Agni"?
11. A robust "Agni" promotes health at how many levels?
12. What are the benefits of fasting?

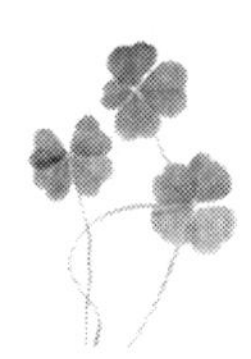

Chapter Seven Review Questions
The Tastes: A Precursor To A Balanced Diet

Test yourself by exploring the following questions:

1. What is taste according to Ayurveda?
2. How many tastes did you know before you read this chapter?
3. How many tastes are there according to Ayurveda?
4. Explain what constitutes taste of a substance in Ayurveda? How can this knowledge be applied? Give examples.
5. What are the most beneficial tastes for Vata dosha?
6. What are the most beneficial tastes for Pitta dosha?
7. What are the most beneficial tastes for Kapha dosha?
8. Why cannot you taste anything when you are sick with the flu?
9. What is a craving in Ayurveda?
10. How would you know if it is a good craving or a bad craving?
11. Which taste is best suited to bringing weight gain and why?
12. Which taste is best for effective weight loss?
13. Which taste is the heaviest and why?
14. Which taste is the lightest and why?
15. Excess of what taste can imbalance Vata?
16. Excess of what taste can calm Pitta?
17. What foods are most astringent?
18. Give examples of bitter tastes?
19. Beans are most prominent in what taste?
20. Are fenugreek seeds astringent, sweet, or bitter?
21. Name one heating spice and explain why?
22. Is licorice bitter or sweet?
23. Name one cooling food?
24. What would be your pick of taste for a cold winter day?

25. What Virya is best for a hot summer day?
26. What is so special about ginger? Are ginger and galangal interchangeable in usage? Explain.
27. Can fruits and dairy products be compatible when used together? Support your answer with example?

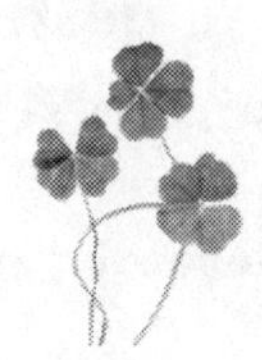

Chapter Eight Review Questions
The Six Stages Of The Digestion Process Congruent To The Six Tastes

Test yourself by exploring the following questions:

1. How many tastes are there?
2. How many stages of digestion does food pass through?
3. What constitutes a balanced diet?
4. An excess of spicy foods affects which part of the digestion process?
5. What foods are best for a Pitta constitution in summer?
6. What foods must a Vata constitution avoid in fall?
7. What is Rasa of foods?
8. What is Virya?
9. How does knowing Virya of a substance or medicinal herb help you? Explain with example.
10. What is Vipaka?
11. How many Vipaka are there?
12. What Virya of substance should a Vata constitution prefer especially during the fall?
13. What dosha is dominant in infancy, and why?
14. Why do infants drool?
15. Drooling in adults could be an indicator of the onset of what disease?
16. In what stage of digestion do the acidic and alkali mix in the intestines?

17. Which enzymes are acidic in nature? Which enzymes are alkaline?
18. What part of food gets digested in the small intestines?
19. What taste is present in the fifth stage of digestion?
20. What happens in the last stage of digestion?
21. Why is it good to scrape your tongue after brushing your teeth in the morning?
22. What effect does "Agni" play on digestion?
23. What health ailments are prevalent when there is an excess of each of the six tastes in one's diet? Give an example for each case (sweet, sour, salty, pungent, bitter, and astringent)?
24. What is the leading cause of poor absorption?
25. How do genetically modified foods (GMOs) affect our body?
26. After which stage does the body generate a false sense of hunger?
27. When is the best time to eat again?
28. Why and how does proper elimination help your health?
29. Considering what you now know of tastes and the digestion process, which taste would be best to add to your diet and why?
30. Is your present diet a balanced diet? Explain why or why not.

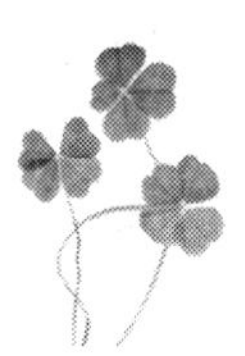

Chapter Nine Review Questions The Wonder Foods That Can Rescue You: Nature's Best Healers

Test yourself by exploring the following questions:

1. How is nourishing food important for our well-being?
2. What constituted the original diet according to Ayurvedic texts?
3. Does choice of food affect our well-being? According to Ayurveda, how many types of foods are there? Give examples to support your answers.
4. Which grain is considered the "King of Grains" and which legume

is the "Queen of Legumes"?

5. How many tastes are there? How many tastes does an amalaki fruits have? Name them. Which tastes is it missing, if any?
6. What is amalaki commonly called?
7. In which Ayurvedic formulations is amalaki one of the important ingredients?
8. Which of the wonder foods would you choose to improve your own digestive fire? Why?
9. What would you recommend to use for a sunburn and why?
10. If an infant in your family is sick with a cold and has congestion in the winter, what would you recommend to improve his condition and why?
11. On a hot summer day, what would your choice of drink be if you were suffering from heat stroke? Why?
12. Which part of the ginger plant is most widely used?
13. What is the foremost taste of amalaki in the mouth? Have you tasted it before? Would you like to?
14. What is post-digestive taste in ginger? How is it different from galangal and why?
15. What would be your choice between ginger and galangal for a person with peptic ulcers? Why?
16. What is a recipe for promoting good digestion?
17. How many flowers do honey bees have to collect nectar from to make one kilogram of honey for us?
18. Is all honey the same? Support your answer.
19. What is the most important benefit credited to amalaki? Did you know about it before you read this book? Would you like to try it out?
20. What is the best sweetener for a kapha constitution and why?
21. What wonder food would you choose for clearing acne and psoriasis? Why?
22. Which food is a "divine elixir"?
23. Which food is a healing panacea?
24. What is the difference between butter as a fat source and "clarified butter" as a fat source? Which one is better and why?
25. Which can stay on the kitchen counter for a longer time without getting rancid – butter or ghee? Why?

26. What is medicated ghee called in Ayurvedic terms?
27. What is the best medicated ghee for mental afflictions?
28. What food choice is best for increasing vitality in an elderly person?
29. What is the best wonder food for supplementing an infant's growth?
30. What is your best friend if you are looking to either shed or gain a few pounds?
31. Which wonder foods will beautify and tone your skin? Why?
32. What do the Europeans do to take care of hard-to-heal wounds?
33. What herb would you mix with aloe to make up a bitter tonic?
34. What wonder food would improve your memory and the health of the nerve cells in your brain?
35. ⋆What are the best wonder foods for a Parkinson's or an Alzheimer's patient? Hint: Both are Vata disorders! What wonder food is the best friend of vata dosha? BONUS MARKS IF YOU GET THIS! It can be more than one.
36. Which wonder food would save you from weak immune deficiency?
37. Name the wonder food that takes on the properties of other foods and boosts their bio-availability and absorbability?
38. Which wonder food will best improve the health of your hair? Explain how. ⋆⋆This is an extra challenge here!
39. What is the body tissues' essence that assimilates food in our body? Health prevails in its presence. What foods can promote its quantity and quality?
40. Which is your lactose-free fat option in your diet – butter or ghee? Why?
41. This food works on thyroid and pituitary glands and ovaries. What is it? Is it safe for a pregnant woman to eat?
42. Is it safe to consume honey that is thick and in a crystallized form? Explain.
43. Presence of this_____________ in saturated fats is found to inhibit tumor growths?
44. What variety of Ghritas best in skin afflictions? Explain and give example.
45. How many honey bees are usually in a beehive?
46. How many flowers do honeybees have to visit to make one kilogram of honey?

47. After reading this chapter, which food would you like to introduce into your diet and why?
48. Which one of these wonder foods had you not heard about before reading this chapter?
49. Which wonder food would you recommend for a cancer or AIDS patient? Why?
50. How has knowing about these wonder foods helped you? Explain reflectively.

APPENDIX I

Ayurvedic Dosha and Food Suggestions: Vata Pacifying Food List

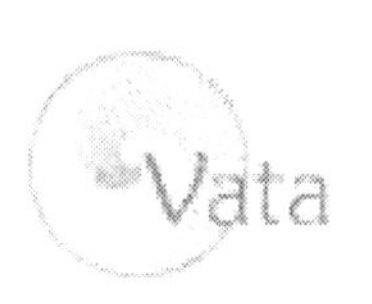

KAPHA TIMES: 6:00 to 10:00 a.m. and p.m.

PITTA TIMES: 10:00 to 2:00 a.m. and p.m.

VATA TIMES: 2:00 to 6:00 a.m. and p.m.

Once you know what your Ayurvedic dosha is, you can balance it by learning what foods support you and what food can further aggravate your dosha.

NOTE:

*** OK in moderation**
**** OK occasionally**!

FRUITS: apricots, avocados, bananas, berries, dates, fresh figs, grapefruit, grapes, kiwis, lemons, mangos, sweet melons, oranges, papaya, peaches, pineapple, plums, strawberries (sweet fruits are pacifying**.)**

AVOID: all dry fruits, raw apple, pears, dry prunes ⋆, dry raisins ⋆ (okay if soaked)

VEGETABLES: avocados, artichokes, asparagus, beets, carrots, cucumbers, green beans, leeks, mustard greens, okra, olives, onions, parsnip (cooked vegetables are most balancing.)

AVOID: raw and frozen vegetables, brocolli, cabbage, cauliflower, celery, eggplants, fresh corn, raw tomatoes (cooked ok), mushrooms, raw peas, peppers, winter squash, white potatoes, kale , raw onions

GRAINS: amaranth, cooked oats, brown rice, basmati white, wild rice, quinoa, wheat

AVOID: barley, bran, yeast breads, buckwheat, corn, dry oats, rice cakes, millet

LEGUMES adzuki beans, red lentils, mung beans, soy cheese, soy milk, tofu

AVOID: black beans, chick peas, kidney beans, miso⋆⋆, pinto beans, soy beans, tempeh

NUTS: all nuts are ok in moderaton; whenever possible soak first

AVOID: peanuts are the most aggravating

SEEDS: sunflower, pumpkin, flax, sesame, chia

AVOID: psyllium

MEATS: beef, dark chicken and turkey, eggs, freshwater fish, seafood, shrimp

AVOID: lamb, mutton, pork, white chicken and turkey, rabbit, venison

HERBS, SPICES, SWEETENERS AND CONDIMENTS: brown rice syrup, honey, maple syrup, molasses, other sweeteners than white sugar, allspice, almond extract, anise, basil, bay leaf, black pepper, caraway, cardamon,carob*, cayenne, chamomile, cinnamon, cloves, coriander, coconut, cumin, dill, fennel, garlic, ginger, mustard, nutmeg, onion, oregano. parsley, peppermint, poppy seeds, rosemary, sage, spearmint, spirulina, tamarind, tarragon, thyme, pickles, salt, seaweed, soy sauce, turmeric, vanilla

AVOID: chocolate, horseradish

OILS: (internal and external use) ghee, sesame, olive (most oils are ok.)

AVOID: flax seed oil

DAIRY: buttermilk, cow's milk, soft cheeses, goat's milk, sweet or spiced yogurts, butter, ghee

AVOID: powdered milks (cow or goat), ice cream, frozen yogurts or fruit yogurts

BEVERAGES: almond milk, apple cider, alcohol (light beer, white sweet wines*), lemonade, orange juice, pineapple juice, hot spiced soy milk

AVOID: hard alcohols and spirits, red wine, apple juice, caffeinated beverages, cranberry juice, iced drinks, cold soy milk, tomato juice

HERBAL TEAS: cinnamon**, fennel, licorice, peppermint, rosehip

AVOID: ginseng, nettle, dandelion, red clover**, yerba mate**

PACIFYING TASTES ARE: sweet, sour, salty

AGGRAVATING TASTES ARE: bitter, pungent, astringent

****These are general guidelines only, cannot make up for a proper ayurvedic consultation to further gear them to one's specific requirements .**

APPENDIX II

Ayurvedic Dosha and Food Suggestions: Pitta Pacifying Food List

KAPHA TIMES: 6:00 to 10:00 a.m. and p.m.

PITTA TIMES: 10:00 to 2:00 a.m. and p.m.

VATA TIMES: 2:00 to 6:00 a.m. and p.m.

Once you know what your Ayurvedic dosha is, you can balance it by learning what foods support you and what food can further aggravate your dosha.

NOTE:

* **OK in moderation**
** **OK occasionally**!

FRUITS: sweet fruits (sweet apples, berries, cherries, oranges, pears, pineapples, plums), dates, figs, purple grapes*, limes, prunes, raisins

AVOID: sour fruits (sour apples, bananas, berries, cherries, oranges, pineapples, plums), grapefruit, green grapes, lemons, peaches

VEGETABLES: (most sweet and bitter vegetables are good) avocados, artichokes, asparagus, cooked beets, broccoli, cabbage, carrots, cooked cauliflower, celery, cucumber, leafy greens, kale, collard, dandelions, aragula, green beans, mushrooms, cooked onions, green peppers, peas, sweet potatoes, white potatoes, most sprouts, squashes, zucchini, brussel sprouts, okra, fresh fennel, parsely, parsnip, lime

AVOID: most pungent kinds, raw beets, fresh corn**, eggplants, mustard greens, raw onions, raw spinach, cooked tomatoes**, hot chilli peppers , lemons

GRAINS: amaranth, barley, bran, granola, quinoa, cooked oats, basmati rice (white and wild), rice cakes, wheat

AVOID: yeast breads, buckwheat, corn, millet, dry oats, brown rice, rye

LEGUMES: black beans, chick peas, kidney beans, pinto beans, all lentils, mung beans, soy beans, soy milk, soy cheese, tempeh*, tofu

AVOID: miso, soy sauce

NUTS: soaked and peeled almonds, fresh coconut

AVOID: no nuts except those suggested above

SEEDS: flax, psyllium, pumpkin*, sunflower, chia

AVOID: sesame, tahini

MEATS: white chicken and turkey, egg whites, freshwater fish, rabbit, shrimp*, venison

AVOID: beef, dark chicken and turkey, egg yolks, sea fish, pork, lamb, mutton

HERBS, SPICES, SWEETENERS AND CONDIMENTS: black pepper*, carob,cinnamon, coriander, cumin, fennel, fresh ginger, saffron, vanilla*, turmeric, seaweed, humus, spearmint, peppermint, dill, wintergreen, barley malt, honey*, rice syrup, natural organic sugar, maple syrup, agave

AVOID: chilli peppers, garlic, dry ginger, horseradish, asafoetida (hing), bay leaf, cloves, ketchup, oregano, nutmeg, cayenne, garlic, mustard seeds, lemons, mayonnaise, onions, pickles, sea salt, sesame seeds, soy sauce, tamari, molasses, white sugar**

OILS: ghee, sunflower, olive (for external use only, coconut oil)

AVOID: corn, apricot, safflower, sesame, almond

DAIRY: butter (unsalted), cottage cheese, mild soft cheeses, ghee, cow's milk, goat's milk, buttermilk

AVOID: salted butter, hard cheeses, feta cheese, sour cream, yogurt

BEVERAGES: dry white wine*, beer, almond milk, apple juice, brewed fresh coffee, orange juice*, pomegranate juice, prune juice, rice milk, soy milk

AVOID: hard spirits, caffeinated drinks, cranberry juice, grapefruit juice, icy drinks, pineapple juice, tomato juice, lemonade, iced tea, chocolate milk

HERBAL TEAS: chamomile, dandelion, licorice, fennel, mint, red clover

AVOID: cinnamon**, ginseng, rosehips**, yerba mate

PACIFYING TASTES: sweet, bitter, astringent

AGGRAVATING TASTES: sour, salty, pungent

****These are general guidelines only, cannot make up for a proper ayurvedic consultation to further gear them to one's specific requirements .**

APPENDIX III

Ayurvedic Dosha and Food Suggestions: Kapha Pacifying Food List

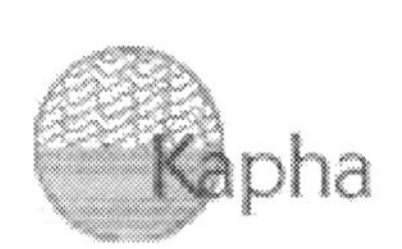

KAPHA TIMES: 6:00 to 10:00 a.m. and p.m.

PITTA TIMES: 10:00 to 2:00 a.m. and p.m.

VATA TIMES: 2:00 to 6:00 a.m. and p.m.

Once you know what your Ayurvedic dosha is, you can balance it by learning what foods support you and what food can further aggravate your dosha.

NOTE:

*** OK in moderation**
**** OK occasionally!**

FRUITS: apples, cherries, dry figs, grapes★, lemons★, limes★, peaches, pears, prunes, raisins, blueberries, blackberries, strawberries★, papaya, mango★

AVOID: sweet and sour fruits, bananas, dates, melons, oranges, pineapples, plums

VEGETABLES: most pungent and bitter vegetables, asparagus, beets greens, broccoli, cabbage, carrots, cauliflower, celery, corn, eggplants, green beans, peppers, okra, kale, collard, arugula, spinach★, mustard greens , mushrooms, onions, peas, peppers, sprouts, winter squash, cooked tomatoes★, horseradish, radishes, turnip, watercress

AVOID: sweet and juicy ones, cucumbers, black/green olives, parsnip★★, pumpkin, summer squash, raw tomatoes, zucchini

GRAINS: amaranth★, barley, bran, buckwheat, quinoa, corn, granola, millet, dry oats, rye, basmati rice★

AVOID: yeast breads, cooked oats, pasta★★, white rice, rice cakes, wheat, spelt, kamut, gluten

LEGUMES: adzuki beans, chick peas, mung beans★, all lentils, dry peas, pinto beans, romano beans, navy beans, soy milk, tempeh, spiced tofu

AVOID: miso, kidney beans, soy beans, soy cheese, soya sauce, and cold tofu

NUTS: charoli or chironji nuts

AVOID: most nuts, almonds★★, coconut★★

SEEDS: flax★, pumpkin★, sunflower★

AVOID: psyllium★★, sesame

MEATS: white chicken and turkey, eggs (poached or boiled only), rabbit, shrimp, venison

AVOID: beef, dark chicken and turkey, sea fish, lamb, mutton, pork

HERBS, SPICES, SWEETENERS AND CONDIMENTS: all heating spices are good, black pepper, black cardamon,carob,cloves, cinnamon, pippali, fenugreek, hot chilli peppers, horseradish, mustard seeds, seaweed★, kelp, basil, oregano, nutmeg, sage, rosemary, poppy seeds, tarragon, thyme, turmeric, scallions, ginger (fresh and dry), garlic, honey (raw unpasteurized), fruit juice concentrates

AVOID: salts, chocolate, lime, mayonnaise, oil pickels, vinegars, (except apple cider vinegar with mother), barley malt, maple syrup, molasses, natural sugar, white sugar

OILS: (for both external and internal usage, use small amounts only) corn, sunflower, mustard, sesame

AVOID: " avoid all oils except exceptions above as noted"

DAIRY: buttermilk★, ghee★, cottage cheese★, unripe cheeses★, skim goat's milk, diluted yogurt only

AVOID: salted butter, no hard cheeses, cow's milk, buffalo milk and cheeses, ice cream, sour cream, creams, fruit yogurt, frozen yogurt

BEVERAGES: dry wines★, apple juice/ cider★, cranberry juice, fresh grain coffee, grape juice, pineapple juice★, pomegranate juice, prune juice, hot spiced soy milk

AVOID: hard liquor, hard beer, sweet wines, almond milk, caffeinated beverages★★, grapefruit juice, iced tea, icy drinks, pops, orange juice, tomato juice, clam juice, rice milk

HERBAL TEAS: black tea, spiced teas, cinnamon, fennel★, yerba mate, peppermint, ginger

AVOID: marshmellow, licorice, rosehips★★

PACIFYING TASTES: pungent, bitter, and astringent

AGGRAVATING TASTES: sweet, sour, and salty

★★These are general guidelines only, cannot make up for a proper ayurvedic consultation to further gear them to one's specific requirements .

APPENDIX IV:
Ayurvedic Constitution Chart

www.ayurvedasoham.com
Ayurvedic Wisdom in Daily Living

OBSERVA-TION	V	P	K	VATA	PITTA	KAPHA
Body size				Slim	Medium	Large
Body Weight				Low	Medium	Overweight
Skin				Thin, Dry, Cold, Rough, Dark	Smooth, Oily, Warm, Rosy	Thick, Oily, Cool, White, Pale
Hair				Dry, Brown, Black, Knotted, Brittle, Thin	Straight, Oily, Blond, Gray, Red, Bald	Thick, Curly, Oily, Wavy, Luxuriant, All colors
Teeth				Protruding, Big, Roomy, Thin gums	Medium, Soft, Tender gums	Healthy, White, Strong gums
Nose				Uneven shape, Deviated Septum	Long, Pointed, Red nose-tip	Short, Round, Button nose
Eyes				Small, Sunken, Dry, Active, Black, Brown, Nervous	Sharp, Bright, Gray, Green, Yellow/Red, Sensitive to light	Big, Beautiful, Blue, Calm, Loving
Nails				Dry, Rough, Brittle, Break easily	Sharp, Flexible, Pink, Lustrous	Thick, Oily, Smooth, Polished
Lips				Dry, Cracked, Black/Brown	Red, Inflamed, Tinged, Yellowish	Smooth, Oily, Pale, Whitish
Chin				Thin, Angular	Tapering	Rounded, Double
Cheeks				Wrinkled, Sunken	Smooth, Flat	Rounded, Plump

OBSERVATION	V	P	K	VATA	PITTA	KAPHA
Neck				Thin, Tall	Medium	Big, Folded
Chest				Flat, Sunken	Moderate	Expanded, Round
Belly				Thin, Flat, Sunken	Moderate	Big, Potbellied
Belly Button				Small, Irregular, Herniated	Oval, Superficial	Big, Deep, Round, Stretched
Hips				Slender, Thin	Moderate	Heavy, Big
Joints				Cold, Cracking	Moderate	Large, Lubricated
Appetite				Irregular, Scanty	Strong, Unbearable	Slow but Steady
Digestion				Irregular, Forms gas	Quick, Causes burning	Prolonged, Forms mucus
Taste, Healthy				Sweet, Sour, Salty	Sweet, Bitter, Astringent	Bitter, Pungent, Astringent
Thirst				Changeable	Surplus	Sparse
Elimination				Constipation	Loose	Thick, Oily, Sluggish
Physical				Hyperactive	Moderate	Sedentary
Mental				Always Active	Moderate	Dull, Slow
Emotions				Anxiety, Fear, Uncertainty	Anger, Hate, Flexible, Jealousy	Calm, Greedy, Determined, Attachment
Faith				Variable, Changeable	Intense, Extremist	Consistent, Deep, Mellow

OBSERVATION	**V**	**P**	**K**	**VATA**	**PITTA**	**KAPHA**
Intellect				Quick but faulty response	Accurate response	Slow, Exact
Recollection				Recent good	Distinct	Slow and sustained
Dreams				Quick, Active, Many, Fearful	Fiery, War, Violence	Lakes, Snow, Romantic
Sleep				Scanty, Broken, Sleeplessness	Little but sound	Deep, Prolonged
Speech				Rapid, Unclear	Sharp, Penetrating	Slow, Monotonous
Financial				Poor, Spends on trifles	Spends money on Luxuries, Education	Rich, Good, Money preserver
TOTAL						

TOTAL EACH

V _____ P_____ K_____

Name: ____

Date: ________________________

CHECK WHAT APPLIES TO YOU THE MOST ACCURATELY THEN TOTAL ALL V, P, & K!

APPENDIX V:
Food Combining Reference Chart

DON'T COMBINE:	WITH FOODS LIKE:
Milk	Bananas, Fish, Meat, Melon, Sour Fruits, Kitchadi, Yeast Bread, Cherries, Yogurt
Melons	Grains, Starch, Fried Foods, Dairy Products
Starches**	Eggs, Tea, Dairy, Bananas, Dates, Persimmons and Most Fruits,
Honey	Cooked on Heat/Mixed in Equal Amount with Ghee
Radishes	Milk, Bananas, Raisins
Nightshades (Tomatoes, Potatoes, Eggplants)	Yogurt, Milk, Melon, Cucumber
Yogurt	Milk, Sour Fruits, Melons
Hot beverages like Tea / Coffee	Meat, Fish, Mangos, Starch, Cheese
Eggs	Milk, Meat, Yogurt, Melons, Cheese, Fish, Bananas
Fruits	With Any Other foods, and especially dairy products
Corn	Dates, Raisins, Bananas
Lemon	Yogurt, Milk, Cucumbers, Tomatoes

APPENDIX VI:

Homemade Ghee ("Clarified Butter") Recipe

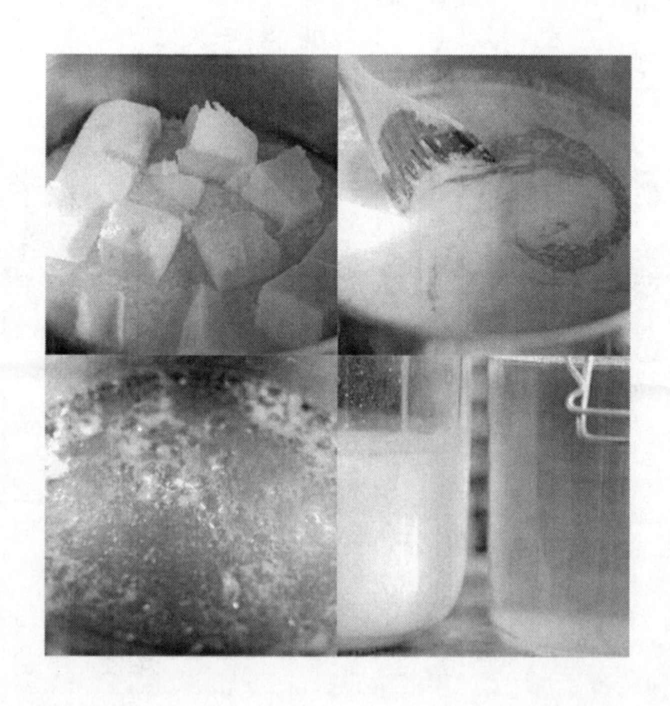

Ingredients and Utensils:

Unsalted Butter – 1 pound brick

Cheesecloth – quadrupled-folded, thick-layered

1 small strainer that can fit on bottle mouth

Mason jar or litre bottle

1 medium stainless steel heavy saucepan

1 wooden spoon

Method:

Boil unsalted butter on low heat in a steel saucepan. Keep stirring with a clean, dry wooden spoon until butter is foamy. Keep butter on a slow boil for 10-15 minutes or until foam subsides, the butter looks clear and is a golden color, and the foam changes to golden brown grits. Strain the clarified butter through a cheesecloth on a small strainer and bottle the golden liquid part. Milk solids left on the cheesecloth can be used in cooking or discarded.

STORAGE: Keep ghee in a glass Mason jar for future use. Once the water in the butter has been properly evaporated, it does not need refrigeration. Take care not to use a wet spoon to take the ghee out of the bottle as it can contaminate your batch. Generally I take a few spoonfuls out to keep in a small dish on the counter for daily use. Make an effort to keep the ghee in the bottle clean and fresh.

CAUTION: Once contaminated, ghee will go rancid fairly quickly.

AYURVEDIC BENEFITS: V ↓ P↓ K ↑

Glossary

A

Aam – the metabolic toxins that result due to improper digestion; it clogs the bodily channels where it lodges and hinders the proper functioning of absorption and assimilation processes in the body

Accredited – that which is officially recognized as meeting the essential requirements

Adipose fat – subcutaneous layer of the fat tissue of the body

Adraka – Common name used for the herb ginger root

Affinity – a natural liking for or an attraction to a person, thing, or an idea; for example, water has an affinity towards gravity and always moves towards it

Agni – The fire element, the second of the five great elements in the body; specifically here it is in reference to the "digestive fire" that helps regulate the body temperature, digestion, absorption, and assimilation processes in the body

Agnivardhak – "Agni" is fire and "vardhak" is the substance that increases fire; applied to foods and herbs it helps ignite the fire element in the body

Ahamkara – The 'I am' feeling, which one associates with day-to-day living; it relates personally to thinking, feeling, and acting

Anabolic – metabolic actions that increase the production of the bodily tissues

Animate – a living thing that grows; or to give life to something

Artava – Female reproductive tissue; closely related to the juice of life (the "rasa dhatu") due to its functional integrity with both the menstruation and lactation processes in females

Assimilate – to take in and incorporate as one's own; to convert food into substances suitable for our bodies to take into its tissues; or to take a thought and absorb its essence within

Asthi – the bone tissue; one of the seven dhatus (bodily tissues) that gives a body a frame that shapes it and provides protection and strength

Atharva Veda – Fourth of the four ancient scriptures of the East Indian holy doctrines; contains all knowledge regarding Ayurveda principles regarding foods, herbs, medicine, and therapy protocols. Sometimes it is referred to as the "UpaVeda" of Ayurveda: the cream nectar of the Atharva Veda

Avila – A cloudy quality, such as confusion or a cloudy perception; it increases kapha and decreases vata and pitta

B

Buddhi – is the individual intelligence; the reasoning capacity of the mind; the intellect

C

Catabolic – any activity that decreases the production of the bodily tissues is catabolic in nature

Chala – the mobile quality; denoted by mobility and changeability, it increases vata and pitta, but decreases kapha

Clairvoyant – an individual, who has the ability to perceive events in the future or beyond the normal sensory reach

Cognition – to understand and differentiate

Cohesive – a quality of sticking together, such as particles of the same substance in one unit

Conducive – making a certain situation or outcome likely or possible

Congestive – any substance that causes congestion or blocking in some part of the body

Congruent – something that is aligning with or coinciding exactly when superimposed

D

Dhatus – the body tissues; Ayurveda defines seven body tissues or dhatus: blood, plasma, muscle, fat, bone, nerve, bone marrow, and the reproductive tissues (both male and female)

Discernment – the quality of being able to differentiate

Drava – the liquid quality that a substance possesses; the fluid quality of water or juices

E

Efficacy – innate power or usefulness of substances

Emesis – cleansing through use of herbs that can encourage vomiting (also called Vamana)

Emollient – a substance having a quality of softening or soothing the skin; to bring about a calming effect

Enumeration – a series of cause and effect applied to the unfolding of a process

Esophagus – the portion of the digestive tube from the mouth to the stomach; general term is the food pipe

Etheric-body – is the subtle body; the vital body and the first or the lowest layer in the "human energy field" or aura; it is said to be in immediate contact with the physical body in order to sustain it and connect it with the "higher bodies"

Embodies – that which gives expression of or gives visible form to an idea, quality, or a feeling

G

Ghritas – In Sanskrit, "Ghrit" means "Ghee" (clarified butter), thus Ghritas are the Ayurvedic medicinal ghee preparations made by infusion with healing herbs; for example, Brahmi Ghrita is ghee made with a Brahmi decoction boiled into the ghee

Gunas – A quality or an attribute; one of the twenty universal attributes; one of the three innate universal qualities in nature (the Sattva, representing the pure light of consciousness; Rajas representing the movement of the process of perception; and Tamas representing darkness and the material sense of this world)

Guru – means the teacher who teaches you about your connection to your higher self; Guru also denotes the heavy quality that is bulky in nature; it increases kapha and decreases vata and pitta

H

Homeostasis – Is a state of balance in the body; derived from the Greek word "homeo", meaning "constant" and "stasis" meaning stable; that which is constantly stable

Hydrophilic – substances that have a strong affinity for water; "hydro" means water and "philic" means affinity; for example, chia seeds and psyllium husk are hydrophilic in nature

I

Inanimate – lifeless, spiritless, lacking perception; an object

Inhabits – that which lives in something, be it person, animal, or a group

Intercellular – meaning activities within one cell

Intracellular – meaning activities around the cells; in between the cell-to-cell function

J

Jathara Agni – the central fire of the digestive system; its prime functions include digestion and assimilation of ingested foods in order to nourish the deeper bodily tissues

K

Kapha – one of the three doshas; the bio energies; made up of the earth and water elements, it is the heaviest of the three doshas; it gives the structural integrity to cell membranes

Kashaya – the astringent taste; made up of the air and the earth elements, it increases vata dosha and decreases pitta and kapha doshas

Kathina – the hard quality; applies to foods like nuts, hardness of cysts and tumors, rigid temperament, etc.; this quality increases vata and kapha and decreases pitta

Katu – the pungent taste; made up of air and fire elements, it increases vata and pitta. but calms the kapha dosha

Khara – the rough quality in things, which represents dryness; it can cause constipation and mal-absorption; it increases vata and decreases pitta and kapha doshas

Kinetic Energy – relates to the energy that a body or a system possesses by virtue of its motion; it is the movement principle

Kledaka kapha – One of the kapha sub-types; it is present in the oral cavity and stomach lining; its prime function is to help in the chewing of ingested foods to make them into liquid form; it is commonly called "mucus" in the mouth and the "gastric mucosal lining" in the stomach; it forms the protective layer in the stomach that protects it from digestive enzymes that are strongly acidic; the fire contained in water

L

Laghu – means a light quality in things; an attribute that signifies lightness or suppleness; it aids digestion and cleansing; vata and pitta possess this quality

Lavana – denotes the salty taste; made up of the fire and water elements, it increases kapha and pitta, but decreases vata dosha

M

Mahad – the Great Cosmic Intelligence Principle; present in the Universe, it is inclusive of individual intelligence, ego, and the mind

Majja – One of the Seven dhatus (bodily tissues); it constitutes the bone marrow, connective tissues, and nerve tissue; associated with the endocrine system and production of red blood cells, its prime role is communication and to fill the hollow spaces inside the bone tissue

Malas – are the body's waste matter; consists of feces, urine, and sweat

Mamsa – One of the Seven dhatus; includes all the muscle, tendon, and cartilage tissues in the body; its functions include movement, protection, giving body its shape, confidence, and strength

Manifestation – an action that shows something; creating with willingness in the heart, we can manifest anything we want in life; a symptom of a disease is its manifestation

Meda dhatu – One of the Seven dhatus; the adipose fat tissue in the body; it represents all fats in the body – be they cholesterol or triglycerides; its prime function includes the lubrication function in all systems of the body

Mimamsa – one of the Six Philosophies (doctrines) of life that Ayurveda incorporates; Mimamsa's proponent was Sage Jaimni; it deals with the understanding of inner reality to better understand outer reality as narrated originally in the Vedas

Mrudu – denotes the soft quality which is delicate; it represents soft things in the body and the mind be it mucus, adipose fat, or tenderness in love; aggravates the kapha and pitta doshas but calming to vata dosha

N

Nyaya – is one of the Six Philosophies (doctrines) of life that Ayurveda incorporates; Nyaya's proponent is Sage Gautama; he deals with gaining knowledge through observation and logic and through using the reasoning power with which we are gifted

O

Ojas – is the end product essence of the foods we intake, kapha in nature, it nourishes all body tissues and improves immunity, strength, and vitality

Omnipotent – the unlimited authority that encompasses everything

Omnipresent – that entity that is present in each aspect of life

Optimal – the most desirable or satisfactory

Osmotic – a process by which molecules of solvent tend to pass through a semi-permeable membrane from a less concentrated solution into a higher concentrated one, thus balancing both sides of the membrane

P

Panchakarma – "Panch" meaning five, "Karma" meaning actions; the five actions in Ayurveda's cleansing program; used to eliminate the excess dosha and metabolic toxins (the Aam) from the body for an overall purification; consists of vomiting therapy (vamana), purgation therapy (virechana), herbal enema therapy (basti with decoction or oils), blood-letting therapy (rakta moksha), and nasal administration therapy (nasya therapy)

Precursor – one that precedes (comes before) something and indicates the approach of another; for example, an immature, unstable dhatu formation is the precursor to the mature, stable dhatu formation

Peristalsis – is the rhythmic contraction of the smooth muscles to propel food through the gastro intestinal tract

Pitta – one of the three doshas; a bio-energy formed by the interaction of the elements of fire and water; it is responsible for the digestion, metabolism, absorption, assimilation, nutrition and maintaining body temperature

Potential Energy – is the energy-possessed by a body or a system by virtue of its position relative to others; it is the hidden potential in a body or a system

Prabhava – is the special effect in substances that just is and cannot be logically explained, but is considered divine in nature

Prakruti – is the primordial matter; the Cosmic Mother, the active principle in the process of "Creation"; it is the innate nature in things, and it symbolizes the constitution of an individual which is the unique combination of the three bio-energies of vata, pitta, and kapha in an individual; it does not change like heat or light in a fire and coolness in the water

Prana – the essence of the air element, without which life cannot be sustained; it is the force behind the cellular intelligence; it governs all communications in the human body; it is the subtle essence of the vata dosha

Pranayama – is a yoga practice signifying the Prana;made up of two Sanskrit words,'prana' the pure subtle essence of vata, and 'yama' meaning to control: therefore Pranayama signifies the systematic controlling of this vital force through this practice, which brings about the healing of the body, mind, and soul

Pruthivi – is Mother Earth or the earth element

Prognosis – is an opinion, based on medical experience, of the likely course a condition will take; a forecast of a likely outcome of a situation

Propagate – to cause to spread or to be transmitted

Purgatives – substances that cause purging of the bowel movement

Q

Qualitative – a measure of things by its quality in size, appearance, value, etc.

Quantitative – a measure of things by its quantity rather than its qualities

R

Rajas – is one of the three universal qualities of the consciousness and/or a substance; it represents the kinetic energy and the active mobile principle

Rajasic – the substances possessing the Rajas quality are called Rajasic in nature; they are sharp, active, mobile; it applies to foods and qualities of the mind

Rakta – the second dhatu; blood tissue; its main function is to maintain life by oxygenation and through the transportation of nutrients throughout the body; it is the most vital fluid in the body and must be protected at all cost

Rasas – means nectar, juice, tastes, joy anything that gives a feeling of satisfaction; it is the subtle essence of the water element

Recessed eyes – meaning deeply seated eyes

Ruksha – is the dry quality; it creates constriction, dehydration, and choking in the body or isolation, fear, and nervousness in the mind

S

Salvation – liberation from ignorance and illusion

Sandra – is the dense quality; foods that are heavy like meats and cheeses; they increase kapha dosha and decrease vata and pitta; it promotes grounding and strength

Sankhya – one of the Six Philosophies Ayurveda incorporates; its proponent is Sage Kapila; it gives Ayurveda the theory of cause and effect in the enumeration process of the cosmic evolution of energy to matter.

The word "Sankhya" relates to the word "sat" meaning "truth" and "khya" meaning "knowledge"; simply it is the knowledge of the Truth

Sattva – One of the three qualities of consciousness and/or substances; it is a pure essence, clear and potential energy that imparts energy to wisdom, understanding, and cognition; it gives rise to mind and senses in Sankhya Philosophy, making up the organic world

Shita – Cool quality; associated with coolness in foods or the mind, for example, cilantro is cool, fear and insensitivity is cool

Shukra – the male reproductive tissue; one of the seven dhatus; semen

Shlakshana – smooth quality; the lubrication function in the body

Snehana – from the word "sneha" meaning loving; all the oil therapies (both internal or external); using oils is associated with love, therefore oil therapies are known as Snehana therapies; it calms the vata dosha

Snigdha – the oily quality; being thick, viscous, and oily in nature; relates to qualities like lubrication, smoothness, love, and compassion; it calms vata while increases pitta and kapha dosha

Static – that which does not move; immobile; denotes dullness, confusion, and darkness

Sthira – the stable quality; deals with support and stability; the skeletal bones and muscles tissue have this quality as they act as support for our body

Sunthi – dry ginger root powder; more heating than the fresh ginger root

T

Tamas – is one of the three universal qualities of consciousness; principle of darkness, ignorance, and inertia; it is responsible for sleep, heaviness, confusion, and decay

Tamasic – substances that carry the tamas quality are tamasic in nature; includes heavy, stale foods and most meats

Tanmatras – are sound, touch, form, taste and smell; these are the subtle energies in the five great elements. Ether represents sound, air represents touch, fire represents form, water represents taste, and earth represents the sense of smell.

Tikshana – the sharp quality, either for foods or the mind; hot chilli peppers are sharp as is the understanding and comprehension of an idea or a theory by the mind

Tikta – the bitter taste; made up of the air and ether elements, it increases vata and decreases both pitta and kapha dosha

Transmute – to change in form or appearance; applies to someone or something

Tridoshas – are the three bio-energies that arise from interaction of the five elements; ether and air elements gave rise to vata dosha, fire and water elements gave rise to pitta dosha, and earth and water elements gave rise to kapha dosha; from "tri" meaning "three and "dosha" meaning an entity that can go out of balance

Triphala – a Ayurvedic herbal preparation; from "tri" meaning "three" and "phala" meaning "fruit"; it is made up of three fruits that are tri-doshic in their benefits: Amalaki (pacify pitta) + Bibhitaki (pacify kapha) + Haritaki (pacify vata)

U

Unctuous – a substance that has a greasy or soapy feel to it

Unleavened – unfermented baked goods or breads that are made without using yeast (instead generally using yogurt or sprouted grains as a leavening agent)

Ushna – the hot quality; this quality in foods helps ignite the digestive fire and improve digestion processes to promote cleansing; it displays as irritability and anger in the mind

V

Vaisheshika – is one of the Six Philosophies (doctrines) of life incorporated by Ayurveda; its proponent is Sage Kanada; it holds to the atomic theory of existence and claims that the entire universe is made up of atoms and that the movement of atoms is governed by the supreme will of The Supreme Being

Vamana – one of the therapies in the Panchkarma protocol; specifically deals with therapeutic vomiting to clear congestion in the lungs; this therapy is most effective in treating coughs, colds, congestion, bronchitis, lymphatic congestion, etc.; it uses emetic herbs like licorice root to bring about Emesis (vomiting)

Vata – is one of the three doshas; produced by the interaction of air and ether elements, it is the lightest of the three doshas that govern all movements in the body and mind

Vayu – air element; second of the five great elements of ether, air, fire, water and earth; it is considered a synonym of vata and can be interchanged with it

Vedanta – "veda" means "knowledge" and "anta" means "in the end", thus is simply "the ending of all knowledge", which is the ultimate goal of the vedas; it is the last of the Six Philosophies of life that Ayurveda incorporates; its proponent is Sage Badarayana; its aim is to end all duality and take one to Oneness

Vedas – the Indian ancient holy scriptures that are a compilation of the teachings of life; there are four vedas: Rig Veda, Sama Veda, Yajur Veda, and Atharva Veda

Vipak – is the post-digestive effect upon consumption in the small intestine, which may be sweet, sour, or pungent in nature

Virechana – from the word "virechan", which means "to take out" or "to expel"; it is one of the therapies in the Panchkarma Protocols; it deals with bringing about purging through the lower pathways; it is especially done to cleanse pitta dosha using various purgative herbs like dandelion root, senna, castor oil, etc.

Virya – is the effect a food or substance leaves initially upon consuming it; it may be either a cooling or heating effect

Viscous – having a thick, sticky consistency that is between solid and liquid, for example, castor oil is highly viscous

Vishada – is the clear quality; relating to substances as well as the mind, for example, water is a clear liquid and it personifies purity and cleansing; in the mind it represents clarity in understanding

Vishvabhesaja – "vishva" means the "universe" and "bhesaja" means "a substance that is a cure-all medicine", thus it means a universal cure-all for all ailments

Y

Yoga – One of the Six Philosophies that Ayurveda incorporates; Sage Patanjali is the proponent of yoga; it personifies the unfolding process of joining one's lower self with one's higher self

Y**ogavahini** – the word "yoga" means "joining" and "vahini" means vehicle; the term applies to substances (food or herbs) that act as a vehicle to transport the healing benefits to the deeper tissues of the subject who consumes it; for example, ghee is yogavahini because it takes on the healing properties of the other foods, herbs, and spices that it is combined with to instigate a healing response in the person who consumes it.

Index of Tables, Flow Charts, Diagrams & Pictures

CPSIA information can be obtained at www.ICGtesting.com
Printed in the USA
LVOW13*0100250314

378731LV00001B/2/P